International Classification of Functioning, Disability and Health

Short version

World Health Organization
Geneva

WHO Library Cataloguing-in-Publication Data

International classification of functioning, disability and health:
ICF Short version.

1.Human development 2.Body constitution 3. Health status
4. Disability evaluation 5.Socioeconomic factors 6.Causality
7.Classification 8.Manuals I.Title: ICF Short version

ISBN 92 4 154544 5   NLM classification: W 15

Contents

ICF

Introduction

1.   Background

This volume contains a concise version of the *International Classification of Functioning, Disability and Health,* known as ICF.[1] The overall aim of the ICF classification is to provide a unified and standard language and framework for the description of health and health-related states. It defines components of health and some health-related components of well-being (such as education and labour). The domains contained in ICF can, therefore, be seen as *health domains* and *health-related domains.* These domains are described from the perspective of the body, the individual and society in two basic lists: (1) Body Functions and Structures; and (2) Activities and Participation.[2] As a classification, ICF systematically groups different domains[3] for a person in a given health condition (e.g. what a person with a disease or disorder does do or can do). *Functioning* is an umbrella term encompassing all body functions, activities and participation; similarly, *disability* serves as an umbrella term for impairments, activity limitations or

---

[1] The text represents a revision of the International Classification of Impairments, Disabilities, and Handicaps (ICIDH), which was first published by the World Health Organization for trial purposes in 1980. Developed after systematic field trials and international consultation over the past five years, it was endorsed by the Fifty-fourth World Health Assembly for international use on 22 May 2001 (resolution WHA54.21).

[2] These terms, which replace the formerly used terms "impairment", "disability" and "handicap", extend the scope of the classification to allow positive experiences to be described. The new terms are further defined in this Introduction and are detailed within the classification. It should be noted that these terms are used with specific meanings that may differ from their everyday usage.

[3] A domain is a practical and meaningful set of related physiological functions, anatomical structures, actions, tasks, or areas of life.

participation restrictions. ICF also lists environmental factors that interact with all these constructs. In this way, it enables the user to record useful profiles of individuals' functioning, disability and health in various domains.

ICF belongs to the "family" of international classifications developed by the World Health Organization (WHO) for application to various aspects of health. The WHO family of international classifications provides a framework to code a wide range of information about health (e.g. diagnosis, functioning and disability, reasons for contact with health services) and uses a standardized common language permitting communication about health and health care across the world in various disciplines and sciences.

In WHO's international classifications, health conditions (diseases, disorders, injuries, etc.) are classified primarily in ICD-10 (shorthand for the International Classification of Diseases, Tenth Revision),[4] which provides an etiological framework. Functioning and disability associated with health conditions are classified in ICF. ICD-10 and ICF are therefore complementary,[5] and users are encouraged to utilize these two members of the WHO family of international classifications together. ICD-10 provides a "diagnosis" of diseases, disorders or other health conditions, and this information is enriched by the additional information given by ICF on functioning.[6] Together,

---

[4] International Statistical Classification of Diseases and Related Health Problems, Tenth Revision, Vols. 1-3. Geneva, World Health Organization, 1992-1994.

[5] It is also important to recognize the overlap between ICD-10 and ICF. Both classifications begin with the body systems. Impairments refer to body structures and functions, which are usually parts of the "disease process" and are therefore also used in the ICD-10. Nevertheless, ICD-10 uses impairments (as signs and symptoms) as parts of a constellation that forms a "disease", or sometimes as reasons for contact with health services, whereas the ICF system uses impairments as problems of body functions and structures associated with health conditions.

information on diagnosis plus functioning provides a broader and more meaningful picture of the health of people or populations, which can then be used for decision-making purposes.

The WHO family of international classifications provides a valuable tool to describe and compare the health of populations in an international context. The information on mortality (provided by ICD-10) and on health outcomes (provided by ICF) may be combined in summary measures of population health for monitoring the health of populations and its distribution, and also for assessing the contributions of different causes of mortality and morbidity.

ICF has moved away from being a "consequence of disease" classification (1980 version) to become a "components of health" classification. "Components of health" identifies the constituents of health, whereas "consequences" focus on the impacts of diseases or other health conditions that may follow as a result. Thus, ICF takes a neutral stand with regard to etiology so that researchers can draw causal inferences using appropriate scientific methods. Similarly, this approach is also different from a "determinants of health" or "risk factors" approach. To facilitate the study of determinants or risk factors, ICF includes a list of environmental factors that describe the context in which individuals live.

---

[6] Two persons with the same disease can have different levels of functioning, and two persons with the same level of functioning do not necessarily have the same health condition. Hence, joint use enhances data quality for medical purposes. Use of ICF should not bypass regular diagnostic procedures. In other uses, ICF may be used alone.

2. Aims of ICF

ICF is a multipurpose classification designed to serve various disciplines and different sectors. Its specific aims can be summarized as follows:

- to provide a scientific basis for understanding and studying health and health-related states, outcomes and determinants;

- to establish a common language for describing health and health-related states in order to improve communication between different users, such as health care workers, researchers, policy-makers and the public, including people with disabilities;

- to permit comparison of data across countries, health care disciplines, services and time;

- to provide a systematic coding scheme for health information systems.

These aims are interrelated, since the need for and uses of ICF require the construction of a meaningful and practical system that can be used by various consumers for health policy, quality assurance and outcome evaluation in different cultures.

2.1 Applications of ICF

Since its publication as a trial version in 1980, ICIDH has been used for various purposes, for example:

- as a statistical tool – in the collection and recording of data (e.g. in population studies and surveys or in management information systems);

- as a research tool – to measure outcomes, quality of life or environmental factors;

- as a clinical tool – in needs assessment, matching treatments with specific conditions, vocational assessment, rehabilitation and outcome evaluation;

- as a social policy tool – in social security planning, compensation systems and policy design and implementation;

- as an educational tool – in curriculum design and to raise awareness and undertake social actions.

Since ICF is inherently a health and health-related classification it is also used by sectors such as insurance, social security, labour, education, economics, social policy and general legislation development, and environmental modification. It has been accepted as one of the United Nations social classifications and is referred to in and incorporates *The Standard Rules on the Equalization of Opportunities for Persons with Disabilities.*[7] Thus ICF provides an appropriate instrument for the implementation of stated international human rights mandates as well as national legislation.

ICF is useful for a broad spectrum of different applications, for example social security, evaluation in managed health care, and population surveys at local, national and international levels. It offers a conceptual framework for information that is applicable to personal health care, including prevention, health promotion, and the improvement of participation by removing or mitigating societal hindrances and encouraging the provision of social supports and facilitators. It is also useful for the study of health care systems, in terms of both evaluation and policy formulation.

---

[7] *The Standard Rules on the Equalization of Opportunities for Persons with Disabilities.* Adopted by the United Nations General Assembly at its 48th session on 20 December 1993 (resolution 48/96). New York, NY, United Nations Department of Public Information, 1994.

3. Properties of ICF

A classification should be clear about what it classifies: its universe, its scope, its units of classification, its organization, and how these elements are structured in terms of their relation to each other. The following sections explain these basic properties of ICF.

3.1 Universe of ICF

ICF encompasses all aspects of human health and some health-relevant components of well-being and describes them in terms of *health domains* and *health-related domains*.[8] The classification remains in the broad context of health and does not cover circumstances that are not health-related, such as those brought about by socioeconomic factors. For example, because of their race, gender, religion or other socioeconomic characteristics people may be restricted in their execution of a task in their current environment, but these are not health-related restrictions of participation as classified in ICF.

There is a widely held misunderstanding that ICF is only about people with disabilities; in fact, it is about *all people*. The health and health-related states associated with all health conditions can be described using ICF. In other words, ICF has universal application.[9]

---

[8] Examples of health domains include seeing, hearing, walking, learning and remembering, while examples of health-related domains include transportation, education and social interactions.

[9] Bickenbach JE, Chatterji S, Badley EM, Üstün TB. Models of disablement, universalism and the ICIDH, *Social Science and Medicine*, 1999, 48:1173-1187.

3.2 Scope of ICF

ICF provides a description of situations with regard to human functioning and its restrictions and serves as a framework to organize this information. It structures the information in a meaningful, interrelated and easily accessible way.

ICF organizes information in two parts. Part 1 deals with Functioning and Disability, while Part 2 covers Contextual Factors. Each part has two components:

1. Components of Functioning and Disability

The **Body** component comprises two classifications, one for functions of body systems, and one for body structures. The chapters in both classifications are organized according to the body systems.

The **Activities and Participation** component covers the complete range of domains denoting aspects of functioning from both an individual and a societal perspective.

2. Components of Contextual Factors

A list of **Environmental Factors** is the first component of Contextual Factors. Environmental factors have an impact on all components of functioning and disability and are organized in sequence from the individual's most immediate environment to the general environment.

Personal Factors is also a component of Contextual Factors but they are not classified in ICF because of the large social and cultural variance associated with them.

The components of Functioning and Disability in Part 1 of ICF can be expressed in two ways. At one end they can be used to indicate problems (e.g. impairment, activity limitation or participation restriction summarized under the umbrella term *disability*); on the other hand they can indicate nonproblematic (i.e. neutral) aspects of health and health-related states summarized under the umbrella term *functioning*).

These components of functioning and disability are interpreted by means of four separate but related *constructs*. These constructs are operationalized by using *qualifiers*. Body functions and structures can be interpreted by means of changes in physiological systems or in anatomical structures. For the Activities and Participation component, two constructs are available: *capacity* and *performance* (see section 4.2).

A person's functioning and disability is conceived as a dynamic interaction[10] between health conditions (diseases, disorders, injuries, traumas, etc.) and contextual factors. As indicate above, Contextual Factors include both personal and environmental factors. ICF includes a comprehensive list of environmental factors as an essential component of the classification. Environmental factors interact with all the components of functioning and disability. The basic construct of the Environmental Factors component is the facilitating or hindering impact of features of the physical, social and attitudinal world.

3.3 Unit of classification

ICF classifies health and health-related states. The unit of classification is, therefore, *categories* within health and health-related domains. It is important to note, therefore, that in ICF persons are not the units of classification; that is, ICF does not classify people, but describes the situation of each person within an array of health or health-related domains. Moreover, the description is always made within the context of environmental and personal factors.

---

[10] This interaction can be viewed as a *process* or a *result* depending on the user.

3.4 Presentation of ICF

ICF is presented in two versions in order to meet the needs of different users for varying levels of detail.

The *full version* of ICF provides classification at four levels of detail. These four levels can be aggregated into a higher-level classification system that includes all the domains at the second level. The *short version*, which is contained in this volume, provides the first two levels of the classification.

4. Overview of ICF components

DEFINITIONS[11]

In the context of health:

Body functions are the physiological functions of body systems (including psychological functions).

Body structures are anatomical parts of the body such as organs, limbs and their components.

Impairments are problems in body function or structure such as a significant deviation or loss.

Activity is the execution of a task or action by an individual.

Participation is involvement in a life situation.

Activity limitations are difficulties an individual may have in executing activities.

Participation restrictions are problems an individual may experience in involvement in life situations.

Environmental factors make up the physical, social and attitudinal environment in which people live and conduct their lives.

---

[11] See also Annex 1, Taxonomic and terminological issues

An overview of these concepts is given in Table 1; they are explained further in operational terms in section 5.1. As the table indicates:

- ICF has two *parts*, each with two *components:*

    Part 1. Functioning and Disability

    (a) Body Functions and Structures

    (b) Activities and Participation

    Part 2. Contextual Factors

    (c) Environmental Factors

    (d) Personal Factors

- Each component can be expressed in both *positive* and *negative* terms.

- Each component consists of various domains and, within each domain, categories, which are the units of classification. Health and health-related states of an individual may be recorded by selecting the appropriate category code or codes and then adding *qualifiers*, which are numeric codes that specify the extent or the magnitude of the functioning or disability in that category, or the extent to which an environmental factor is a facilitator or barrier.

Table 1. An overview of ICF

	Part 1: Functioning and Disability		Part 2: Contextual Factors	
Components	Body Functions and Structures	Activities and Participation	Environmental Factors	Personal Factors
Domains	Body functions Body structures	Life areas (tasks, actions)	External influences on functioning and disability	Internal influences on functioning and disability
Constructs	Change in body functions (physiological) Change in body structures (anatomical)	Capacity Executing tasks in a standard environment Performance Executing tasks in the current environment	Facilitating or hindering impact of features of the physical, social, and attitudinal world	Impact of attributes of the person
Positive aspect	Functional and structural integrity	Activities Participation	Facilitators	not applicable
	Functioning			
Negative aspect	Impairment	Activity limitation Participation restriction	Barriers / hindrances	not applicable
	Disability			

4.1 Body Functions and Structures and impairments

Definitions: **Body *functions*** *are the physiological functions of body systems (including psychological functions).*

Body *structures* *are anatomical parts of the body such as organs, limbs and their components.*

Impairments *are problems in body function or structure as a significant deviation or loss.*

(1)   Body functions and body structures are classified in two different sections. These two classifications are designed for use in parallel. For example, body functions include basic human senses such as "seeing functions" and their structural correlates exist in the form of "eye and related structures".

(2)   "Body" refers to the human organism as a whole; hence it includes the brain and its functions, i.e. the mind. Mental (or psychological) functions are therefore subsumed under body functions.

(3)   Body functions and structures are classified according to body systems; consequently, body structures are not considered as organs.[12]

---

[12] Although organ level was mentioned in the 1980 version of ICIDH, the definition of an "organ" is not clear. The eye and ear are traditionally considered as organs; however, it is difficult to identify and define their boundaries, and the same is true of extremities and internal organs. Instead of an approach by "organ", which implies the existence of an entity or unit within the body, ICF replaces this term with "body structure".

(4)   Impairments of structure can involve an anomaly, defect, loss or other significant deviation in body structures. Impairments have been conceptualized in congruence with biological knowledge at the level of tissues or cells and at the subcellular or molecular level. For practical reasons, however, these levels are not listed.[13] The biological foundations of impairments have guided the classification and there may be room for expanding the classification at the cellular or molecular levels. For medical users, it should be noted that impairments are not the same as the underlying pathology, but are the manifestations of that pathology.

(5)   Impairments represent a deviation from certain generally accepted population standards in the biomedical status of the body and its functions, and definition of their constituents is undertaken primarily by those qualified to judge physical and mental functioning according to these standards.

(6)   Impairments can be temporary or permanent; progressive, regressive or static; intermittent or continuous. The deviation from the population norm may be slight or severe and may fluctuate over time. These characteristics are captured in further descriptions, mainly in the codes, by means of qualifiers after the point.

(7)   Impairments are not contingent on etiology or how they are developed; for example, loss of vision or a limb may arise from a genetic abnormality or an injury. The presence of an impairment necessarily implies a cause; however, the cause may not be sufficient to explain the resulting impairment.

---

[13] Thus impairments coded using the full version of ICF should be detectable or noticeable by others or the person concerned by direct observation or by inference from observation.

Also, when there is an impairment, there is a dysfunction in body functions or structures, but this may be related to any of the various diseases, disorders or physiological states.

(8) Impairments may be part or an expression of a health condition, but do not necessarily indicate that a disease is present or that the individual should be regarded as sick.

(9) Impairments are broader and more inclusive in scope than disorders or diseases; for example, the loss of a leg is an impairment of body structure, but not a disorder or a disease.

(10) Impairments may result in other impairments; for example, a lack of muscle power may impair movement functions, heart functions may relate to deficit in respiratory functions, and impaired perception may relate to thought functions.

(11) Some categories of the Body Functions and Structures component and the ICD-10 categories seem to overlap, particularly with regard to symptoms and signs. However, the purposes of the two classifications are different. ICD-10 classifies symptoms in special chapters to document morbidity or service utilization, whereas ICF shows them as part of the body functions, which may be used for prevention or identifying patients' needs. Most importantly, in ICF the Body Functions and Structures classification is intended to be used along with the Activities and Participation categories.

(12) Impairments are classified in the appropriate categories using defined identification criteria (e.g. as present or absent according to a threshold level). These criteria are the same for body functions and structures. They are: (a) loss or lack; (b) reduction; (c) addition or excess; and (d) deviation. Once an impairment is present, it may be scaled in terms of its severity using the generic qualifier in the ICF.

(13) Environmental factors interact with body functions, as in the interactions between air quality and breathing, light and seeing, sounds and hearing, distracting stimuli and attention, ground texture and balance, and ambient temperature and body temperature regulation.

4.2 Activities and Participation /activity limitations and participation restrictions

Definitions: *Activity is the execution of a task or action by an individual.*

     Participation is involvement in a life situation.

     Activity limitations are difficulties an individual may have in executing activities.

     Participation restrictions are problems an individual may experience in involvement in life situations.

(1) The domains for the Activities and Participation component are given in a *single list* that covers the full range of life areas (from basic learning or watching to composite areas such as interpersonal interactions or employment). The component can be used to denote activities (a) or participation (p) or both. The domains of this component are qualified by the two qualifiers of *performance* and *capacity*. Hence the information gathered from the list provides a data matrix that has no overlap or redundancy (see Table 2).

Table 2. Activities and Participation: information matrix

	Domains	Qualifiers	
		Performance	Capacity
d1	Learning and applying knowledge		
d2	General tasks and demands		
d3	Communication		
d4	Mobility		
d5	Self-care		
d6	Domestic life		
d7	Interpersonal interactions and relationships		
d8	Major life areas		
d9	Community, social and civic life		

(2) The *performance* qualifier describes what an individual does in his or her current environment. Because the current environment includes a societal context, performance can also be understood as "involvement in a life situation" or "the lived experience" of people in the actual context in which they live.[14] This context includes the environmental factors – all aspects of the physical, social and attitudinal

---

[14] The definition of "participation" brings in the concept of involvement. Some proposed definitions of "involvement" incorporate taking part, being included or engaged in an area of life, being accepted, or having access to needed resources. Within the information matrix in Table 2 the only possible indicator of participation is coding through performance. This does not mean that participation is automatically equated with performance. The concept of involvement should also be distinguished from the subjective experience of involvement (the sense of "belonging"). Users who wish to code involvement separately should refer to the coding guidelines in Annex 2.

world which can be coded using the Environmental Factors component.

(3) The *capacity* qualifier describes an individual's ability to execute a task or an action. This construct aims to indicate the highest probable level of functioning that a person may reach in a given domain at a given moment. To assess the full ability of the individual, one would need to have a "standardized" environment to neutralize the varying impact of different environments on the ability of the individual. This standardized environment may be: (a) an actual environment commonly used for capacity assessment in test settings; or (b) in cases where this is not possible, an assumed environment which can be thought to have a uniform impact. This environment can be called a "uniform" or "standard" environment. Thus, capacity reflects the environmentally adjusted ability of the individual. This adjustment has to be the same for all persons in all countries to allow for international comparisons. The features of the uniform or standard environment can be coded using the Environmental Factors classification. The gap between capacity and performance reflects the difference between the impacts of current and uniform environments, and thus provides a useful guide as to what can be done to the environment of the individual to improve performance.

(4) Both capacity and performance qualifiers can further be used with and without assistive devices or personal assistance. While neither devices nor personal assistance eliminate the impairments, they may remove limitations on functioning in specific domains. This type of coding is particularly useful to identify how much the functioning of the individual would be limited without the assistive devices (see coding guidelines in Annex 2)

(5)   Difficulties or problems in these domains can arise when
      there is a qualitative or quantitative alteration in the way in
      which an individual carries out these domain functions.
      Limitations or *restrictions* are assessed against a generally
      accepted population standard. The standard or norm
      against which an individual's capacity and performance is
      compared is that of an individual without a similar health
      condition (disease, disorder or injury, etc.). The limitation
      or restriction records the discordance between the observed
      and the expected performance. The expected performance
      is the population norm, which represents the experience of
      people without the specific health condition. The same
      norm is used in the capacity qualifier so that one can infer
      what can be done to the environment of the individual to
      enhance performance.

(6)   A problem with performance can result directly from the
      social environment, even when the individual has no
      impairment. For example, an individual who is HIV-
      positive without any symptoms or disease, or someone with
      a genetic predisposition to a certain disease, may exhibit no
      impairments or may have sufficient capacity to work, yet
      may not do so because of the denial of access to services,
      discrimination or stigma.

(7)   It is difficult to distinguish between "Activities" and
      "Participation" on the basis of the domains in the Activities
      and Participation component. Similarly, differentiating
      between "individual" and "societal" perspectives on the
      basis of domains has not been possible given international
      variation and differences in the approaches of professionals
      and theoretical frameworks. Therefore, ICF provides a
      single list that can be used, if users so wish, to differentiate
      activities and participation in their own operational ways.
      There are four possible ways of doing so:

(a)   to designate some domains as activities and others as participation, not allowing any overlap;

(b)   same as (a) above, but allowing partial overlap;

(c)   to designate all detailed domains as activities and the broad category headings as participation;

(d)   to use all domains as both activities and participation.

4.3 Contextual Factors

Contextual Factors represent the complete background of an individual's life and living. They include two components: Environmental Factors and Personal Factors – which may have an impact on the individual with a health condition and that individual's health and health-related states.

Environmental factors make up the physical, social and attitudinal environment in which people live and conduct their lives. The factors are external to individuals and can have a positive or negative influence on the individual's performance as a member of society, on the individual's capacity or on the individual's body function or structure.

(1)   Environmental factors are organized in the classification to focus on two different levels:

(a)   *Individual* – in the immediate environment of the individual, including settings such as home, workplace and school. Included at this level are the physical and material features of the environment that an individual comes face to face with, as well as direct contact with others such as family, acquaintances, peers and strangers.

(b) *Societal* – formal and informal social structures, services and overarching approaches or systems in the community or society that have an impact on individuals. This level includes organizations and services related to the work environment, community activities, government agencies, communication and transportation services, and informal social networks as well as laws, regulations, formal and informal rules, attitudes and ideologies.

(2) Environmental factors interact with the components of Body Functions and Structures and Activities and Participation. For each component, the nature and extent of that interaction may be elaborated by future scientific work. Disability is characterized as the outcome or result of a complex relationship between an individual's health condition and personal factors, and of the external factors that represent the circumstances in which the individual lives. Because of this relationship, different environments may have a very different impact on the same individual with a given health condition. An environment with barriers, or without facilitators, will restrict the individual's performance; other environments that are more facilitating may increase that performance. Society may hinder an individual's performance because either it creates barriers (e.g. inaccessible buildings) or it does not provide facilitators (e.g. unavailability of assistive devices).

Personal factors are the particular background of an individual's life and living, and comprise features of the individual that are not part of a health condition or health states. These factors may include gender, race, age, other health conditions, fitness, lifestyle, habits, upbringing, coping styles, social background, education, profession, past and current experience (past life events and concurrent events), overall behaviour pattern and character style, individual psychological assets and other characteristics, all or any of which may play a role in disability at any level. Personal factors are not classified in ICF. However, they are included in Fig. 1 to show their contribution, which may have an impact on the outcome of various interventions.

5. Model of Functioning and Disability

5.1 Process of functioning and disability

As a classification, ICF does not model the "process" of functioning and disability. It can be used, however, to describe the process by providing the means to map the different constructs and domains. It provides a multi-perspective approach to the classification of functioning and disability as an interactive and evolutionary process. It provides the building blocks for users who wish to create models and study different aspects of this process. In this sense, ICF can be seen as a language: the texts that can be created with it depend on the users, their creativity and their scientific orientation. In order to visualize the current understanding of interaction of various components, the diagram presented in Fig. 1 may be helpful.[15]

---

[15] ICF differs substantially from the 1980 version of ICIDH in the depiction of the interrelations between functioning and disability. It should be noted that any diagram is likely to be incomplete and prone to misrepresentation because of the complexity of interactions in a multidimensional model. The model is drawn to illustrate multiple interactions. Other depictions indicating other important foci in the process are certainly possible. Interpretations of interactions between different components and constructs may also vary (for example, the impact of environmental factors on body functions certainly differs from their impact on participation).

Fig. 1. Interactions between the components of ICF

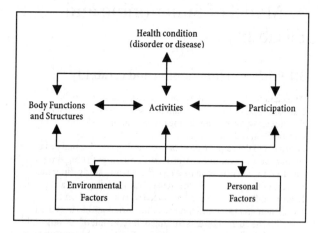

In this diagram, an individual's functioning in a specific domain is an interaction or complex relationship between the health condition and contextual factors (i.e. environmental and personal factors). There is a dynamic interaction among these entities: interventions in one entity have the potential to modify one or more of the other entities. These interactions are specific and not always in a predictable one-to-one relationship. The interaction works in two directions; the presence of disability may even modify the health condition itself. To infer a limitation in capacity from one or more impairments, or a restriction of performance from one or more limitations, may often seem reasonable. It is important, however, to collect data on these constructs independently and thereafter explore associations and causal links between them. If the full health experience is to be described, all components are useful. For example, one may:

- have impairments without having capacity limitations (e.g. a disfigurement in leprosy may have no effect on a person's capacity);

- have performance problems and capacity limitations without evident impairments (e.g. reduced performance in daily activities associated with many diseases);

- have performance problems without impairments or capacity limitations (e.g. an HIV-positive individual, or an ex-patient recovered from mental illness, facing stigmatization or discrimination in interpersonal relations or work);

- have capacity limitations without assistance, and no performance problems in the current environment (e.g. an individual with mobility limitations may be provided by society with assistive technology to move around);

- experience a degree of influence in a reverse direction (e.g. lack of use of limbs can cause muscle atrophy; institutionalization may result in loss of social skills).

The scheme shown in Fig. 1 demonstrates the role that contextual factors (i.e. environmental and personal factors) play in the process. These factors interact with the individual with a health condition and determine the level and extent of the individual's functioning. Environmental factors are extrinsic to the individual (e.g. the attitudes of the society, architectural characteristics, the legal system) and are classified in the Environmental Factors classification. Personal Factors, on the other hand, are not classified in the current version of ICF. They include gender, race, age, fitness, lifestyle, habits, coping styles and other such factors. Their assessment is left to the user, if needed.

5.2 Medical and social models

A variety of conceptual models[16] has been proposed to understand and explain disability and functioning. These may be expressed in a dialectic of "medical model" versus "social model". The *medical model* views disability as a problem of the person, directly caused by disease, trauma or other health condition, which requires medical care provided in the form of individual treatment by professionals. Management of the disability is aimed at cure or the individual's adjustment and behaviour change. Medical care is viewed as the main issue, and at the political level the principal response is that of modifying or reforming health care policy. The *social model* of disability, on the other hand, sees the issue mainly as a socially created problem, and basically as a matter of the full integration of individuals into society. Disability is not an attribute of an individual, but rather a complex collection of conditions, many of which are created by the social environment. Hence the management of the problem requires social action, and it is the collective responsibility of society at large to make the environmental modifications necessary for the full participation of people with disabilities in all areas of social life. The issue is therefore an attitudinal or ideological one requiring social change, which at the political level becomes a question of human rights. For this model disability is a political issue.

ICF is based on an integration of these two opposing models. In order to capture the integration of the various perspectives of functioning, a "biopsychosocial" approach is used. Thus, ICF attempts to achieve a synthesis, in order to provide a coherent view of different perspectives of health from a biological, individual and social perspective.

---

[16] The term "model" here means construct or paradigm, which differs from the use of the term in the previous section.

6. Use of ICF

ICF is a classification of human functioning and disability. It systematically groups health and health-related domains. Within each component, domains are further grouped according to their common characteristics (such as their origin, type, or similarity) and ordered in a meaningful way. The classification is organized according to a set of principles (see Annex 1). These principles refer to the interrelatedness of the levels and the hierarchy of the classification (sets of levels). However, some categories in ICF are arranged in a non-hierarchical manner, with no ordering but as equal members of a branch.

The following are structural features of the classification that have a bearing on its use.

(1)   ICF gives standard operational definitions of the health and health-related domains as opposed to "vernacular" definitions of health. These definitions describe the essential attributes of each domain (e.g. qualities, properties, and relationships) and contain information as to what is included and excluded in each domain. The definitions contain commonly used anchor points for assessment so that they can be translated into questionnaires. Conversely, results from existing assessment instruments can be coded in ICF terms. For example, "seeing functions" are defined in terms of functions of sensing form and contour, from varying distances, using one or both eyes, so that the severity of difficulties of vision can be coded at mild, moderate, severe or total levels in relation to these parameters.

(2)   ICF uses an alphanumeric system in which the letters b, s, d and e are used to denote Body Functions, Body Structures, Activities and Participation, and Environmental Factors.

These letters are followed by a numeric code that starts with the chapter number (one digit), followed by the second level (two digits), and the third and fourth levels (one digit each).

(3) ICF categories are "nested" so that broader categories are defined to include more detailed subcategories of the parent category. (For example, Chapter 4 in the Activities and Participation component, on Mobility, includes separate categories on standing, sitting, walking, carrying items, and so on). The short (concise) version covers two levels, whereas the full (detailed) version extends to four levels. The short version and full version codes are in correspondence, and the short version can be aggregated from the full version.

(4) Any individual may have a range of codes at each level. These may be independent or interrelated.

(5) The ICF codes are only complete with the presence of a *qualifier*, which denotes a magnitude of the level of health (e.g. severity of the problem). Qualifiers are coded as one, two or more numbers after a point (or *separator*). Use of any code should be accompanied by at least one qualifier. Without qualifiers, codes have no inherent meaning.

(6) The first qualifier for Body Functions and Structures, the performance and capacity qualifiers for Activities and Participation, and the first qualifier for Environmental Factors all describe the extent of problems in the respective component.

(7) All three components classified in ICF (Body Functions and Structures, Activities and Participation, and Environmental Factors) are quantified using the same generic scale. Having a problem may mean an impairment, limitation, restriction or barrier depending on the construct. Appropriate

qualifying words as shown in brackets below should be chosen according to the relevant classification domain (where xxx stands for the second-level domain number). For this quantification to be used in a universal manner, assessment procedures need to be developed through research. Broad ranges of percentages are provided for those cases in which calibrated assessment instruments or other standards are available to quantify the impairment, capacity limitation, performance problem or barrier. For example, when "no problem" or "complete problem" is specified the coding has a margin of error of up to 5%. "Moderate problem" is defined as up to half of the time or half the scale of total difficulty. The percentages are to be calibrated in different domains with reference to relevant population standards as percentiles.

xxx.0 NO problem	(none, absent, negligible,…)	0-4 %
xxx.1 MILD problem	(slight, low,…)	5-24 %
xxx.2 MODERATE problem	(medium, fair,...)	25-49 %
xxx.3 SEVERE problem	(high, extreme, …)	50-95 %
xxx.4 COMPLETE problem	(total,…)	96-100 %
xxx.8 not specified		
xxx.9 not applicable		

(8)   In the case of environmental factors, this first qualifier can be used to denote either the extent of positive effects of the environment, i.e. facilitators, or the extent of negative effects, i.e. barriers. Both use the same 0-4 scale, but to denote facilitators the point is replaced by a plus sign: for example e110+2. Environmental Factors can be coded (a) in relation to each construct individually, or (b) overall, without reference to any individual construct. The first option is preferable, since it identifies the impact and attribution more clearly.

(9)   For different users, it might be appropriate and helpful to add other kinds of information to the coding of each item. There are a variety of additional qualifiers that could be

useful. Table 3 sets out the details of the qualifiers for each component as well as suggested additional qualifiers to be developed.

(10) The descriptions of health and health-related domains refer to their use at a given moment (i.e. as a snapshot). However, use at multiple time points is possible to describe a trajectory over time and process.

(11) In ICF, a person's health and health-related states are given an array of codes that encompass the two parts of the classification. Thus the maximum number of codes per person can be 34 at the one-digit level (8 body functions, 8 body structures, 9 performance and 9 capacity codes). Similarly, for the two-level items the total number of codes is 362. At more detailed levels, these codes number up to 1424 items. In real-life applications of ICF, a set of 3 to 18 codes may be adequate to describe a case with two-level (three-digit) precision. Generally the more detailed four-level version is used for specialist services (e.g. rehabilitation outcomes, geriatrics), whereas the two-level classification can be used for surveys and clinical outcome evaluation.

Further coding guidelines are presented in Annex 2. Users are strongly recommended to obtain training in the use of the classification through WHO and its network of collaborating centres.

Table 3. Qualifiers

Components	First qualifier	Second qualifier
Body Functions (b)	Generic qualifier with the negative scale used to indicate the extent or magnitude of an impairment Example: b168.3 to indicate a severe impairment in specific mental functions of language	None
Body Structures (s)	Generic qualifier with the negative scale used to indicate the extent or magnitude of an impairment Example: s730.3 to indicate a severe impairment of the upper extremity	Used to indicate the nature of the change in the respective body structure: 0 no change in structure 1 total absence 2 partial absence 3 additional part 4 aberrant dimensions 5 discontinuity 6 deviating position 7 qualitative changes in structure, including accumulation of fluid 8 not specified 9 not applicable Example: s730.32 to indicate the partial absence of the upper extremity

Components	First qualifier	Second qualifier
Activities and Participation (d)	Performance Generic qualifier Problem in the person's current environment Example: d5101.1_ to indicate mild difficulty with bathing the whole body with the use of assistive devices that are available to the person in his or her current environment	Capacity Generic qualifier Limitation without assistance Example: d5101._2 to indicate moderate difficulty with bathing the whole body; implies that there is moderate difficulty without the use of assistive devices or personal help
Environmental Factors (e)	Generic qualifier, with negative and positive scale, to denote extent of barriers and facilitators respectively Example: e130.2 to indicate that products for education are a moderate barrier. Conversely, e130+2 would indicate that products for education are a moderate facilitator	None

54th World Health Assembly endorsement of ICF for international use

The resolution WHA54.21 reads as follows:

The Fifty-fourth World Health Assembly,

1.   ENDORSES the second edition of the International Classification of Impairments, Disabilities and Handicaps (ICIDH), with the title International Classification of Functioning, Disability and Health, henceforth referred to in short as ICF;

2.   URGES Member States to use ICF in their research, surveillance and reporting as appropriate, taking into account specific situations in Member States and, in particular, in view of possible future revisions;

3.   REQUESTS the Director-General to provide support to Member States, at their request, in making use of ICF.

ICF

One-Level
Classification

List of chapter headings
in the classification

Body functions

Body structures

Chapter 6   Structures related to the genitourinary and
             reproductive systems
Chapter 7   Structures related to movement
Chapter 8   Skin and related structures

Activities and participation

Chapter 1   Learning and applying knowledge
Chapter 2   General tasks and demands
Chapter 3   Communication
Chapter 4   Mobility
Chapter 5   Self-care
Chapter 6   Domestic life
Chapter 7   Interpersonal interactions and relationships
Chapter 8   Major life areas
Chapter 9   Community, social and civic life

Environmental factors

Chapter 1   Products and technology
Chapter 2   Natural environment and human-made
             changes to environment
Chapter 3   Support and relationships
Chapter 4   Attitudes
Chapter 5   Services, systems and policies

ICF

Two-Level classification

List of chapter headings
and first branching level
in the classification

BODY FUNCTIONS

Chapter 1 Mental functions

Global mental functions (b110-b139)
b110   Consciousness functions
b114   Orientation functions
b117   Intellectual functions
b122   Global psychosocial functions
b126   Temperament and personality functions
b130   Energy and drive functions
b134   Sleep functions
b139   Global mental functions, other specified and unspecified

Specific mental functions (b140-b189)
b140   Attention functions
b144   Memory functions
b147   Psychomotor functions
b152   Emotional functions
b156   Perceptual functions
b160   Thought functions
b164   Higher-level cognitive functions
b167   Mental functions of language
b172   Calculation functions
b176   Mental function of sequencing complex movements
b180   Experience of self and time functions
b189   Specific mental functions, other specified and unspecified
b198   Mental functions, other specified
b199   Mental functions, unspecified

Chapter 2 Sensory functions and pain

Seeing and related functions (b210-b229)
b210   Seeing functions
b215   Functions of structures adjoining the eye
b220   Sensations associated with the eye and adjoining structures
b229   Seeing and related functions, other specified and unspecified

Hearing and vestibular functions (b230-b249)
b230   Hearing functions
b235   Vestibular functions
b240   Sensations associated with hearing and vestibular function
b249   Hearing and vestibular functions, other specified and unspecified

Additional sensory functions (b250-b279)
b250   Taste function
b255   Smell function
b260   Proprioceptive function
b265   Touch function
b270   Sensory functions related to temperature and other stimuli
b279   Additional sensory functions, other specified and unspecified

Pain (b280-b289)
b280   Sensation of pain
b289   Sensation of pain, other specified and unspecified
b298   Sensory functions and pain, other specified
b299   Sensory functions and pain, unspecified

Chapter 3 Voice and speech functions

b310   Voice functions
b320   Articulation functions
b330   Fluency and rhythm of speech functions
b340   Alternative vocalization functions
b398   Voice and speech functions, other specified
b399   Voice and speech functions, unspecified

Chapter 4 Functions of the cardiovascular, haematological, immunological and respiratory systems

Functions of the cardiovascular system (b410-b429)

b410   Heart functions
b415   Blood vessel functions
b420   Blood pressure functions
b429   Functions of the cardiovascular system, other specified and unspecified

Functions of the haematological and immunological systems (b430-b439)

b430   Haematological system functions
b435   Immunological system functions
b439   Functions of the haematological and immunological systems, other specified and unspecified

Functions of the respiratory system (b440-b449)

b440   Respiration functions
b445   Respiratory muscle functions
b449   Functions of the respiratory system, other specified and unspecified

Additional functions and sensations of the cardiovascular and respiratory systems (b450-b469)

b450   Additional respiratory functions
b455   Exercise tolerance functions
b460   Sensations associated with cardiovascular and respiratory functions
b469   Additional functions and sensations of the cardiovascular and respiratory systems, other specified and unspecified
b498   Functions of the cardiovascular, haematological, immunological and respiratory systems, other specified
b499   Functions of the cardiovascular, haematological, immunological and respiratory systems, unspecified

Chapter 5   Functions of the digestive, metabolic and endocrine systems

Functions related to the digestive system (b510-b539)

b510   Ingestion functions
b515   Digestive functions
b520   Assimilation functions
b525   Defecation functions
b530   Weight maintenance functions
b535   Sensations associated with the digestive system
b539   Functions related to the digestive system, other specified and unspecified

Functions related to metabolism and the endocrine system (b540-b559)

b540   General metabolic functions
b545   Water, mineral and electrolyte balance functions
b550   Thermoregulatory functions
b555   Endocrine gland functions
b559   Functions related to metabolism and the endocrine system, other specified and unspecified

b598   Functions of the digestive, metabolic and endocrine
        systems, other specified
b599   Functions of the digestive, metabolic and endocrine
        systems, unspecified

Chapter 6 Genitourinary and reproductive functions

Urinary functions (b610-b639)

b610   Urinary excretory functions
b620   Urination functions
b630   Sensations associated with urinary functions
b639   Urinary functions, other specified and unspecified

Genital and reproductive functions (b640-b679)

b640   Sexual functions
b650   Menstruation functions
b660   Procreation functions
b670   Sensations associated with genital and reproductive
        functions
b679   Genital and reproductive functions, other specified and
        unspecified
b698   Genitourinary and reproductive functions, other
        specified
b699   Genitourinary and reproductive functions, unspecified

Chapter 7 Neuromusculoskeletal and movement-related functions

Functions of the joints and bones (b710-b729)

b710   Mobility of joint functions
b715   Stability of joint functions
b720   Mobility of bone functions
b729   Functions of the joints and bones, other specified and
        unspecified

Muscle functions (b730-b749)

b730 Muscle power functions
b735 Muscle tone functions
b740 Muscle endurance functions
b749 Muscle functions, other specified and unspecified

Movement functions (b750-b789)

b750 Motor reflex functions
b755 Involuntary movement reaction functions
b760 Control of voluntary movement functions
b765 Involuntary movement functions
b770 Gait pattern functions
b780 Sensations related to muscles and movement functions
b789 Movement functions, other specified and unspecified
b798 Neuromusculoskeletal and movement-related functions, other specified
b799 Neuromusculoskeletal and movement-related functions, unspecified

Chapter 8 Functions of the skin and related structures

Functions of the skin (b810-b849)

b810 Protective functions of the skin
b820 Repair functions of the skin
b830 Other functions of the skin
b840 Sensation related to the skin
b849 Functions of the skin, other specified and unspecified

Functions of the hair and nails (b850-b869)

b850 Functions of hair
b860 Functions of nails
b869 Functions of the hair and nails, other specified and unspecified

b898   Functions of the skin and related structures, other
       specified
b899   Functions of the skin and related structures, unspecified

BODY STRUCTURES

Chapter 1 Structures of the nervous system
s110   Structure of brain
s120   Spinal cord and related structures
s130   Structure of meninges
s140   Structure of sympathetic nervous system
s150   Structure of parasympathetic nervous system
s198   Structure of the nervous system, other specified
s199   Structure of the nervous system, unspecified

Chapter 2 The eye, ear and related structures
s210   Structure of eye socket
s220   Structure of eyeball
s230   Structures around eye
s240   Structure of external ear
s250   Structure of middle ear
s260   Structure of inner ear
s298   Eye, ear and related structures, other specified
s299   Eye, ear and related structures, unspecified

Chapter 3 Structures involved in voice and speech
s310   Structure of nose
s320   Structure of mouth
s330   Structure of pharynx
s340   Structure of larynx
s398   Structures involved in voice and speech, other specified
s399   Structures involved in voice and speech, unspecified

Chapter 4 Structures of the cardiovascular, immunological and respiratory systems

s410   Structure of cardiovascular system
s420   Structure of immune system
s430   Structure of respiratory system
s498   Structures of the cardiovascular, immunological and respiratory systems, other specified
s499   Structures of the cardiovascular, immunological and respiratory systems, unspecified

Chapter 5 Structures related to the digestive, metabolic and endocrine systems

s510   Structure of salivary glands
s520   Structure of oesophagus
s530   Structure of stomach
s540   Structure of intestine
s550   Structure of pancreas
s560   Structure of liver
s570   Structure of gall bladder and ducts
s580   Structure of endocrine glands
s598   Structures related to the digestive, metabolic and endocrine systems, other specified
s599   Structures related to the digestive, metabolic and endocrine systems, unspecified

Chapter 6 Structures related to the genitourinary and reproductive systems

s610   Structure of urinary system
s620   Structure of pelvic floor
s630   Structure of reproductive system
s698   Structures related to the genitourinary and reproductive systems, other specified
s699   Structures related to the genitourinary and reproductive systems, unspecified

Chapter 7 Structures related to movement

s710   Structure of head and neck region
s720   Structure of shoulder region
s730   Structure of upper extremity
s740   Structure of pelvic region
s750   Structure of lower extremity
s760   Structure of trunk
s770   Additional musculoskeletal structures related to movement
s798   Structures related to movement, other specified
s799   Structures related to movement, unspecified

Chapter 8 Skin and related structures

s810   Structure of areas of skin
s820   Structure of skin glands
s830   Structure of nails
s840   Structure of hair
s898   Skin and related structures, other specified
s899   Skin and related structures, unspecifed

ACTIVITIES AND PARTICIPATION

Chapter 1 Learning and applying knowledge

Purposeful sensory experiences (d110-d129)
d110 Watching
d115 Listening
d120 Other purposeful sensing
d129 Purposeful sensory experiences, other specified and
        unspecified

Basic learning (d130-d159)
d130 Copying
d135 Rehearsing
d140 Learning to read
d145 Learning to write
d150 Learning to calculate
d155 Acquiring skills
d159 Basic learning, other specified and unspecified

Applying knowledge (d160-d179)
d160 Focusing attention
d163 Thinking
d166 Reading
d170 Writing
d172 Calculating
d175 Solving problems
d177 Making decisions
d179 Applying knowledge, other specified and unspecified
d198 Learning and applying knowledge, other specified
d199 Learning and applying knowledge, unspecified

Chapter 2 General tasks and demands

d210 Undertaking a single task
d220 Undertaking multiple tasks
d230 Carrying out daily routine
d240 Handling stress and other psychological demands
d298 General tasks and demands, other specified
d299 General tasks and demands, unspecified

Chapter 3 Communication

Communicating - receiving (d310-d329)

d310 Communicating with - receiving - spoken messages
d315 Communicating with - receiving - nonverbal messages
d320 Communicating with - receiving - formal sign language messages
d325 Communicating with - receiving - written messages
d329 Communicating - receiving, other specified and unspecified

Communicating - producing (d330-d349)

d330 Speaking
d335 Producing nonverbal messages
d340 Producing messages in formal sign language
d345 Writing messages
d349 Communication - producing, other specified and unspecified

Conversation and use of communication devices and techniques (d350-d369)

d350 Conversation
d355 Discussion
d360 Using communication devices and techniques
d369 Conversation and use of communication devices and techniques, other specified and unspecified
d398 Communication, other specified

d399 Communication, unspecified

Chapter 4 Mobility

Changing and maintaining body position (d410-d429)

d410 Changing basic body position
d415 Maintaining a body position
d420 Transferring oneself
d429 Changing and maintaining body position, other specified and unspecified

Carrying, moving and handling objects (d430-d449)

d430 Lifting and carrying objects
d435 Moving objects with lower extremities
d440 Fine hand use
d445 Hand and arm use
d449 Carrying, moving and handling objects, other specified and unspecified

Walking and moving (d450-d469)

d450 Walking
d455 Moving around
d460 Moving around in different locations
d465 Moving around using equipment
d469 Walking and moving, other specified and unspecified

Moving around using transportation (d470-d489)

d470 Using transportation
d475 Driving
d480 Riding animals for transportation
d489 Moving around using transportation, other specified and unspecified
d498 Mobility, other specified
d499 Mobility, unspecified

Chapter 5 Self-care

d510 Washing oneself
d520 Caring for body parts
d530 Toileting
d540 Dressing
d550 Eating
d560 Drinking
d570 Looking after one's health
d598 Self-care, other specified
d599 Self-care, unspecified

Chapter 6 Domestic life

Acquisition of necessities (d610-d629)

d610 Acquiring a place to live
d620 Acquisition of goods and services
d629 Acquisition of necessities, other specified and unspecified

Household tasks (d630-d649)

d630 Preparing meals
d640 Doing housework
d649 Household tasks, other specified and unspecified

Caring for household objects and assisting others (d650-d669)

d650 Caring for household objects
d660 Assisting others
d669 Caring for household objects and assisting others, other specified and unspecified
d698 Domestic life, other specified
d699 Domestic life, unspecified

Chapter 7 Interpersonal interactions and relationships

General interpersonal interactions (d710-d729)

d710   Basic interpersonal interactions
d720   Complex interpersonal interactions
d729   General interpersonal interactions, other specified and unspecified

Particular interpersonal relationships (d730-d779)

d730   Relating with strangers
d740   Formal relationships
d750   Informal social relationships
d760   Family relationships
d770   Intimate relationships
d779   Particular interpersonal relationships, other specified and unspecified
d798   Interpersonal interactions and relationships, other specified
d799   Interpersonal interactions and relationships, unspecified

Chapter 8 Major life areas

Education (d810-d839)

d810   Informal education
d815   Preschool education
d820   School education
d825   Vocational training
d830   Higher education
d839   Education, other specified and unspecified

Work and employment (d840-d859)

d840   Apprenticeship (work preparation)
d845   Acquiring, keeping and terminating a job
d850   Remunerative employment
d855   Non-remunerative employment

d859   Work and employment, other specified and unspecified

Economic life (d860-d879)
d860   Basic economic transactions
d865   Complex economic transactions
d870   Economic self-sufficiency
d879   Economic life, other specified and unspecified
d898   Major life areas, other specified
d899   Major life areas, unspecified

Chapter 9 Community, social and civic life
d910   Community life
d920   Recreation and leisure
d930   Religion and spirituality
d940   Human rights
d950   Political life and citizenship
d998   Community, social and civic life, other specified
d999   Community, social and civic life, unspecified

ENVIRONMENTAL FACTORS

e245 Time-related changes
e250 Sound
e255 Vibration
e260 Air quality
e298 Natural environment and human-made changes to environment, other specified
e299 Natural environment and human-made changes to environment, unspecified

Chapter 3 Support and relationships

e310 Immediate family
e315 Extended family
e320 Friends
e325 Acquaintances, peers colleagues, neighbours and community members
e330 People in positions of authority
e335 People in subordinate positions
e340 Personal care providers and personal assistants
e345 Strangers
e350 Domesticated animals
e355 Health professionals
e360 Health-related professionals
e398 Support and relationships, other specified
e399 Support and relationships, unspecified

Chapter 4 Attitudes

e410 Individual attitudes of immediate family members
e415 Individual attitudes of extended family members
e420 Individual attitudes of friends
e425 Individual attitudes of acquaintances, peers colleagues, neighbours and community members
e430 Individual attitudes of people in positions of authority
e435 Individual attitudes of people in subordinate positions
e440 Individual attitudes of personal care providers and personal assistants

e445   Individual attitudes of strangers
e450   Individual attitudes of health professionals
e455   Individual attitudes of health-related professionals
e460   Societal attitudes
e465   Social norms, practices and ideologies
e498   Attitudes, other specified
e499   Attitudes, unspecified

Chapter 5 Services, systems and policies

e510   Services, systems and policies for the production of consumer goods
e515   Architecture and construction services, systems and policies
e520   Open space planning services, systems and policies
e525   Housing services, systems and policies
e530   Utilities services, systems and policies
e535   Communication services, systems and policies
e540   Transportation services, systems and policies
e545   Civil protection services, systems and policies
e550   Legal services, systems and policies
e555   Associations and organizational services, systems and policies
e560   Media services, systems and policies
e565   Economic services, systems and policies
e570   Social security services, systems and policies
e575   General social support services, systems and policies
e580   Health services, systems and policies
e585   Education and training services, systems and policies
e590   Labour and employment services, systems and policies
e595   Political services, systems and policies
e598   Services, systems and policies, other specified
e599   Services, systems and policies, unspecified

ICF

Detailed classification with definitions

All second level categories with their definitions,
inclusions and exclusions

BODY FUNCTIONS

Definitions: **Body functions** are the physiological functions of body systems (including psychological functions).

Impairments are problems in body function or structure as a significant deviation or loss.

Qualifier

Generic qualifier with the negative scale, used to indicate the extent or magnitude of an impairment:

xxx.0 NO impairment	(none, absent, negligible,...)	0-4 %
xxx.1 MILD impairment	(slight, low,...)	5-24 %
xxx.2 MODERATE impairment	(medium, fair,...)	25-49 %
xxx.3 SEVERE impairment	(high, extreme, ...)	50-95 %
xxx.4 COMPLETE impairment	(total,...)	96-100 %
xxx.8 not specified		
xxx.9 not applicable		

Broad ranges of percentages are provided for those cases in which calibrated assessment instruments or other standards are available to quantify the impairment in body function. For example, when "no impairment" or "complete impairment" in body function is coded, this scaling may have margin of error of up to 5%. "Moderate impairment" is generally up to half of the scale of total impairment. The percentages are to be calibrated in different domains with reference to population standards as percentiles. For this quantification to be used in a uniform manner, assessment procedures need to be developed through research.

For a further explanation of coding conventions in ICF, refer to Annex 2.

Chapter 1
Mental functions

This chapter is about the functions of the brain: both global mental functions, such as consciousness, energy and drive, and specific mental functions, such as memory, language and calculation mental functions.

Global mental functions (b110-b139)

b 110   **Consciousness functions**
General mental functions of the state of awareness and alertness, including the clarity and continuity of the wakeful state.

Inclusions: functions of the state, continuity and quality of consciousness; loss of consciousness, coma, vegetative states, fugues, trance states, possession states, drug-induced altered consciousness, delirium, stupor

Exclusions: orientation functions (b114); energy and drive functions (b130); sleep functions (b134)

b 114   **Orientation functions**
General mental functions of knowing and ascertaining one's relation to self, to others, to time and to one's surroundings.

Inclusions: functions of orientation to time, place and person; orientation to self and others; disorientation to time, place and person

Exclusions: consciousness functions (b110); attention functions (b140); memory functions (b144)

b 117   **Intellectual functions**
General mental functions, required to understand and constructively integrate the various mental functions, including all cognitive functions and their development over the life span.

Inclusions: functions of intellectual growth; intellectual retardation, mental retardation, dementia

Exclusions: memory functions (b144); thought functions (b160); higher-level cognitive functions (b164)

b 122   **Global psychosocial functions**
General mental functions, as they develop over the life span, required to understand and constructively integrate the mental functions that lead to the formation of the interpersonal skills needed to establish reciprocal social interactions, in terms of both meaning and purpose.

Inclusion: such as in autism

b126 **Temperament and personality functions**
General mental functions of constitutional disposition
of the individual to react in a particular way to
situations, including the set of mental characteristics
that makes the individual distinct from others.

*Inclusions: functions of extraversion, introversion,
agreeableness, conscientiousness, psychic and emotional
stability, and openness to experience; optimism; novelty
seeking; confidence; trustworthiness*

*Exclusions: intellectual functions (b117); energy and
drive functions (b130); psychomotor functions (b147);
emotional functions (b152)*

b130 **Energy and drive functions**
General mental functions of physiological and
psychological mechanisms that cause the individual to
move towards satisfying specific needs and general
goals in a persistent manner.

*Inclusions: functions of energy level, motivation,
appetite, craving (including craving for substances that
can be abused), and impulse control*

*Exclusions: consciousness functions (b110);
temperament and personality functions (b126); sleep
functions (b134); psychomotor functions (b147);
emotional functions (b152)*

b134 **Sleep functions**
General mental functions of periodic, reversible and selective physical and mental disengagement from one's immediate environment accompanied by characteristic physiological changes.

Inclusions: functions of amount of sleeping, and onset, maintenance and quality of sleep; functions involving the sleep cycle, such as in insomnia, hypersomnia and narcolepsy

Exclusions: consciousness functions (b110); energy and drive functions (b130); attention functions (b140); psychomotor functions (b147)

b139 **Global mental functions, other specified and unspecified**

Specific mental functions (b140-b189)

b140 **Attention functions**
Specific mental functions of focusing on an external stimulus or internal experience for the required period of time.

Inclusions: functions of sustaining attention, shifting attention, dividing attention, sharing attention; concentration; distractibility

Exclusions: consciousness functions (b110); energy and drive functions (b130); sleep functions (b134); memory functions (b144); psychomotor functions (b147); perceptual functions (b156)

b144 **Memory functions**
Specific mental functions of registering and storing information and retrieving it as needed.

Inclusions: functions of short-term and long-term memory, immediate, recent and remote memory; memory span; retrieval of memory; remembering; functions used in recalling and learning, such as in nominal, selective and dissociative amnesia

Exclusions: consciousness functions (b110); orientation functions (b114); intellectual functions (b117); attention functions (b140); perceptual functions (b156); thought functions (b160); higher-level cognitive functions (b164); mental functions of language (b167); calculation functions (b172)

b 147   Psychomotor functions
Specific mental functions of control over both motor
and psychological events at the body level.

*Inclusions: functions of psychomotor control, such as
psychomotor retardation, excitement and agitation,
posturing, catatonia, negativism, ambitendency,
echopraxia and echolalia; quality of psychomotor
function*

*Exclusions: consciousness functions (b110); orientation
functions (b114); intellectual functions (b117); energy
and drive functions (b130); attention functions (b140);
mental functions of language (b167); mental functions
of sequencing complex movements (b176)*

b 152   Emotional functions
Specific mental functions related to the feeling and
affective components of the processes of the mind.

*Inclusions: functions of appropriateness of emotion,
regulation and range of emotion; affect; sadness,
happiness, love, fear, anger, hate, tension, anxiety, joy,
sorrow; lability of emotion; flattening of affect*

*Exclusions: temperament and personality functions
(b126); energy and drive functions (b130)*

b156 **Perceptual functions**
Specific mental functions of recognizing and interpreting sensory stimuli.

Inclusions: functions of auditory, visual, olfactory, gustatory, tactile and visuospatial perception, such as hallucination or illusion

Exclusions: consciousness functions (b110); orientation functions (b114); attention functions (b140); memory functions (b144); mental functions of language (b167); seeing and related functions (b210-b229); hearing and vestibular functions (b230-b249); additional sensory functions (b250-b279)

b160 **Thought functions**
Specific mental functions related to the ideational component of the mind.

Inclusions: functions of pace, form, control and content of thought; goal-directed thought functions, non-goal directed thought functions; logical thought functions, such as pressure of thought, flight of ideas, thought block, incoherence of thought, tangentiality, circumstantiality, delusions, obsessions and compulsions

Exclusions: intellectual functions (b117); memory functions (b144); psychomotor functions (b147); perceptual functions (b156); higher-level cognitive functions (b164); mental functions of language (b167); calculation functions (b172)

b164 **Higher-level cognitive functions**

Specific mental functions especially dependent on the frontal lobes of the brain, including complex goal-directed behaviours such as decision-making, abstract thinking, planning and carrying out plans, mental flexibility, and deciding which behaviours are appropriate under what circumstances; often called executive functions.

Inclusions: functions of abstraction and organization of ideas; time management, insight and judgement; concept formation, categorization and cognitive flexibility

Exclusions: memory functions (b144); thought functions (b160); mental functions of language (b167); calculation functions (b172)

b167 **Mental functions of language**

Specific mental functions of recognizing and using signs, symbols and other components of a language.

Inclusions: functions of reception and decryption of spoken, written or other forms of language such as sign language; functions of expression of spoken, written or other forms of language; integrative language functions, spoken and written, such as involved in receptive, expressive, Broca's, Wernicke's and conduction aphasia

Exclusions: attention functions (b140); memory functions (b144); perceptual functions (b156); thought functions (b160); higher-level cognitive functions (b164); calculation functions (b172); mental functions of complex movements (b176); Chapter 2 Sensory Functions and Pain; Chapter 3 Voice and Speech Functions

b 172 **Calculation functions**
Specific mental functions of determination, approximation and manipulation of mathematical symbols and processes.

Inclusions: functions of addition, subtraction, and other simple mathematical calculations; functions of complex mathematical operations

Exclusions: attention functions (b140); memory functions (b144); thought functions (b160); higher-level cognitive functions (b164); mental functions of language (b167)

b 176 **Mental function of sequencing complex movements**
Specific mental functions of sequencing and coordinating complex, purposeful movements.

Inclusions: impairments such as in ideation, ideomotor, dressing, oculomotor and speech apraxia

Exclusions: psychomotor functions (b147); higher-level cognitive functions (b164); Chapter 7 Neuromusculoskeletal and Movement-Related Functions

b 180 **Experience of self and time functions**
Specific mental functions related to the awareness of one's identity, one's body, one's position in the reality of one's environment and of time.

Inclusions: functions of experience of self, body image and time

b 189 Specific mental functions, other specified and unspecified

b 198 Mental functions, other specified

b 199 Mental functions, unspecified

Chapter 2

Sensory functions and pain

This chapter is about the functions of the senses, seeing, hearing, tasting and so on, as well as the sensation of pain.

Seeing and related functions (b210-b229)

b210   **Seeing functions**
Sensory functions relating to sensing the presence of light and sensing the form, size, shape and colour of the visual stimuli.

Inclusions: visual acuity functions; visual field functions; quality of vision; functions of sensing light and colour, visual acuity of distant and near vision, monocular and binocular vision; visual picture quality; impairments such as myopia, hypermetropia, astigmatism, hemianopia, colour-blindness, tunnel vision, central and peripheral scotoma, diplopia, night blindness and impaired adaptability to light

Exclusion: perceptual functions (b156)

b215   **Functions of structures adjoining the eye**
Functions of structures in and around the eye that
facilitate seeing functions.

*Inclusions: functions of internal muscles of the eye,
eyelid, external muscles of the eye, including voluntary
and tracking movements and fixation of the eye,
lachrymal glands, accommodation, pupillary reflex;
impairments such as in nystagmus, xerophthalmia and
ptosis*

*Exclusions: seeing functions (b210); Chapter 7
Neuromusculoskeletal and Movement-related Functions*

b220   **Sensations associated with the eye and adjoining
structures**
Sensations of tired, dry and itching eye and related
feelings.

*Inclusions: feelings of pressure behind the eye, of
something in the eye, eye strain, burning in the eye; eye
irritation*

Exclusion: sensation of pain (b280)

b229   **Seeing and related functions, other specified and
unspecified**

Hearing and vestibular functions (b230-b249)

b230   **Hearing functions**
Sensory functions relating to sensing the presence of sounds and discriminating the location, pitch, loudness and quality of sounds.

Inclusions: functions of hearing, auditory discrimination, localization of sound source, lateralization of sound, speech discrimination; impairments such as deafness, hearing impairment and hearing loss

Exclusions: perceptual functions (b156) and mental functions of language (b167)

b235   **Vestibular functions**
Sensory functions of the inner ear related to position, balance and movement.

Inclusions: functions of position and positional sense; functions of balance of the body and movement

Exclusion: sensation associated with hearing and vestibular functions (b240)

b240   **Sensations associated with hearing and vestibular function**
Sensations of dizziness, falling, tinnitus and vertigo.

Inclusions: sensations of ringing in ears, irritation in ear, aural pressure, nausea associated with dizziness or vertigo

Exclusions: vestibular functions (b235); sensation of pain (b280)

b 249   Hearing and vestibular functions, other specified
             and unspecified

Additional sensory functions (b250-b279)

b 250   Taste function
             Sensory functions of sensing qualities of bitterness,
             sweetness, sourness and saltiness.

             *Inclusions: gustatory functions; impairments such as
             ageusia and hypogeusia*

b 255   Smell function
             Sensory functions of sensing odours and smells.

             *Inclusions: olfactory functions; impairments such as
             anosmia or hyposmia*

b 260   Proprioceptive function
             Sensory functions of sensing the relative position of
             body parts.

             Inclusions: functions of statesthesia and kinaesthesia

             *Exclusions: vestibular functions (b235); sensations
             related to muscles and movement functions (b780)*

b 265 **Touch function**
Sensory functions of sensing surfaces and their texture or quality.

Inclusions: functions of touching, feeling of touch; impairments such as numbness, anaesthesia, tingling, paraesthesia and hyperaesthesia

Exclusions: sensory functions related to temperature and other stimuli (b270)

b 270 **Sensory functions related to temperature and other stimuli**
Sensory functions of sensing temperature, vibration, pressure and noxious stimulus.

Inclusions: functions of being sensitive to temperature, vibration, shaking or oscillation, superficial pressure, deep pressure, burning sensation or a noxious stimulus

Exclusions: touch functions (b265); sensation of pain (b280)

b 279 **Additional sensory functions, other specified and unspecified**

Pain (b280-b289)

b 280   **Sensation of pain**
Sensation of unpleasant feeling indicating potential or actual damage to some body structure.

Inclusions: sensations of generalized or localized pain, in one or more body part, pain in a dermatome, stabbing pain, burning pain, dull pain, aching pain; impairments such as myalgia, analgesia and hyperalgesia

b 289   Sensation of pain, other specified and unspecified

b 298   Sensory functions and pain, other specified

b 299   Sensory functions and pain, unspecified

Chapter 3
Voice and speech functions

This chapter is about the functions of producing sounds and speech.

b 310 **Voice functions**
Functions of the production of various sounds by the passage of air through the larynx.

Inclusions: functions of production and quality of voice; functions of phonation, pitch, loudness and other qualities of voice; impairments such as aphonia, dysphonia, hoarseness, hypernasality and hyponasality

Exclusions: mental functions of language (b167); articulation functions (b320)

b 320 **Articulation functions**
Functions of the production of speech sounds.

Inclusions: functions of enunciation, articulation of phonemes; spastic, ataxic, flaccid dysarthria; anarthria

Exclusions: mental functions of language (b167); voice functions (b310)

b 330 **Fluency and rhythm of speech functions**
Functions of the production of flow and tempo of speech.

Inclusions: functions of fluency, rhythm, speed and melody of speech; prosody and intonation; impairments such as stuttering, stammering, cluttering, bradylalia and tachylalia

Exclusions: mental functions of language (b167); voice functions (b310); articulation functions (b320)

b 340 **Alternative vocalization functions**
Functions of the production of other manners of vocalization.

Inclusions: functions of the production of notes and range of sounds, such as in singing, chanting, babbling and humming; crying aloud and screaming

Exclusions: mental functions of language (b167); voice functions (b310); articulation functions (b320); fluency and rhythm of speech functions (b330)

b 398 **Voice and speech functions, other specified**

b 399 **Voice and speech functions, unspecified**

Chapter 4
Functions of the cardio-vascular, haematological, immunological and respiratory systems

This chapter is about the functions involved in the cardiovascular system (functions of the heart and blood vessels), the haematological and immunological systems (functions of blood production and immunity), and the respiratory system (functions of respiration and exercise tolerance).

Functions of the cardiovascular system (b410-b429)

b410   **Heart functions**
Functions of pumping the blood in adequate or required amounts and pressure throughout the body.

Inclusions: functions of heart rate, rhythm and output; contraction force of ventricular muscles; functions of heart valves; pumping the blood through the pulmonary circuit; dynamics of circulation to the heart; impairments such as tachycardia, bradycardia and irregular heart beatand as in heart failure, cardiomyopathy, myocarditis,and coronary insufficiency

Exclusions: blood vessel functions (b415); blood pressure functions (b420); exercise tolerance functions (b455)

b415 **Blood vessel functions**
Functions of transporting blood throughout the body.

Inclusions: functions of arteries, capillaries and veins; vasomotor function; functions of pulmonary arteries, capillaries and veins; functions of valves of veins; impairments such as in blockage or constriction of arteries; atherosclerosis, arteriosclerosis, thromboembolism and varicose veins

Exclusions: heart functions (b410); blood pressure functions (b420); haematological system functions (b430); exercise tolerance functions (b455)

b420 **Blood pressure functions**
Functions of maintaining the pressure of blood within the arteries.

Inclusions: functions of maintenance of blood pressure; increased and decreased blood pressure; impairments such as in hypotension, hypertension and postural hypotension

Exclusions: heart functions (b410); blood vessel functions (b415); exercise tolerance functions (b455)

b429 **Functions of the cardiovascular system, other specified and unspecified**

Functions of the haematological and immunological systems (b430-b439)

b 430   **Haematological system functions**
Functions of blood production, oxygen and metabolite carriage, and clotting.

Inclusions: functions of the production of blood and bone marrow; oxygen-carrying functions of blood; blood-related functions of spleen; metabolite-carrying functions of blood; clotting; impairments such as anaemia, haemophilia and other clotting dysfunctions

Exclusions: functions of the cardiovascular system (b410-b429); immunological system functions (b435); exercise tolerance functions (b455)

b 435   **Immunological system functions**
Functions of the body related to protection against foreign substances, including infections, by specific and non-specific immune responses.

Inclusions: immune response (specific and non-specific); hypersensitivity reactions; functions of lymphatic vessels and nodes; functions of cell-mediated immunity, antibody-mediated immunity; response to immunization; impairments such as in autoimmunity, allergic reactions, lymphadenitis and lymphoedema

Exclusion: haematological system functions (b430)

b 439   **Functions of the haematological and immunological systems, other specified and unspecified**

Functions of the respiratory system (b440-b449)

b 440   **Respiration functions**
Functions of inhaling air into the lungs, the exchange of gases between air and blood, and exhaling air.

Inclusions: functions of respiration rate, rhythm and depth; impairments such as apnoea, hyperventilation, irregular respiration, paradoxical respiration, and brochial spasm, and as in pulmonary emphysema

Exclusions: respiratory muscle functions (b445); additional respiratory functions (b450); exercise tolerance functions (b455)

b 445   **Respiratory muscle functions**
Functions of the muscles involved in breathing.

Inclusions: functions of thoracic respiratory muscles; functions of the diaphragm; functions of accessory respiratory muscles

Exclusions: respiration functions (b440); additional respiratory functions (b450); exercise tolerance functions (b455)

b 449   **Functions of the respiratory system, other specified and unspecified**

Additional functions and sensations of the cardiovascular and respiratory systems (b450-b469)

b 450 **Additional respiratory functions**
Additional functions related to breathing, such as coughing, sneezing and yawning.

Inclusions: functions of blowing, whistling and mouth breathing

b 455 **Exercise tolerance functions**
Functions related to respiratory and cardiovascular capacity as required for enduring physical exertion.

Inclusions: functions of physical endurance, aerobic capacity, stamina and fatiguability

Exclusions: functions of the cardiovascular system (b410-b429); haematological system functions (b430); respiration functions (b440); respiratory muscle functions (b445); additional respiratory functions (b450)

b 460 **Sensations associated with cardiovascular and respiratory functions**
Sensations such as missing a heart beat, palpitation and shortness of breath.

Inclusions: sensations of tightness of chest, feelings of irregular beat, dyspnoea, air hunger, choking, gagging and wheezing

Exclusion: sensation of pain (b280)

b469   Additional functions and sensations of the cardiovascular and respiratory systems, other specified and unspecified

b498   Functions of the cardiovascular, haematological, immunological and respiratory systems, other specified

b499   Functions of the cardiovascular, haematological, immunological and respiratory systems, unspecified

Chapter 5
Functions of the digestive, metabolic and endocrine systems

This chapter is about the functions of ingestion, digestion and elimination, as well as functions involved in metabolism and the endocrine glands.

Functions related to the digestive system (b510-b539)

b510 **Ingestion functions**

Functions related to taking in and manipulating solids or liquids through the mouth into the body.

Inclusions: functions of sucking, chewing and biting, manipulating food in the mouth, salivation, swallowing, burping, regurgitation, spitting and vomiting; impairments such as dysphagia, aspiration of food, aerophagia, excessive salivation, drooling and insufficient salivation

Exclusion: sensations associated with digestive system (b535)

b515 **Digestive functions**
Functions of transporting food through the gastrointestinal tract, breakdown of food and absorption of nutrients.

Inclusions: functions of transport of food through the stomach, peristalsis; breakdown of food, enzyme production and action in stomach and intestines; absorption of nutrients and tolerance to food; impairments such as in hyperacidity of stomach, malabsorption, intolerance to food, hypermotility of intestines, intestinal paralysis, intestinal obstruction and decreased bile production

Exclusions: ingestion functions (b510); assimilation functions (b520); defecation functions (b525); sensations associated with the digestive system (b535)

b520 **Assimilation functions**
Functions by which nutrients are converted into components of the living body.

Inclusion: functions of storage of nutrients in the body

Exclusions: digestive functions (b515); defecation functions (b525); weight maintenance functions (b530); general metabolic functions (b540)

b 525 **Defecation functions**
Functions of elimination of wastes and undigested food as faeces and related functions.

Inclusions: functions of elimination, faecal consistency, frequency of defecation; faecal continence, flatulence; impairments such as constipation, diarrhoea, watery stool and anal sphincter incompetence or incontinence

Exclusions: digestive functions (b515); assimilation functions (b520); sensations associated with the digestive system (b535)

b 530 **Weight maintenance functions**
Functions of maintaining appropriate body weight, including weight gain during the developmental period.

Inclusions: functions of maintenance of acceptable Body Mass Index (BMI); and impairments such as underweight, cachexia, wasting, overweight, emaciation and such as in primary and secondary obesity

Exclusions: assimilation functions (b520); general metabolic functions (b540); endocrine gland functions (b555)

b535   **Sensations associated with the digestive system**
Sensations arising from eating, drinking and related
digestive functions.

*Inclusions: sensations of nausea, feeling bloated, and the
feeling of abdominal cramps; fullness of stomach, globus
feeling, spasm of stomach, gas in stomach and heartburn*

*Exclusions: sensation of pain (b280); ingestion functions
(b510); digestive functions (b515); defecation functions
(b525)*

b539   **Functions related to the digestive system, other
specified and unspecified**

Functions related to metabolism and the endocrine system (b540-b559)

b540   **General metabolic functions**
Functions of regulation of essential components of the
body such as carbohydrates, proteins and fats, the
conversion of one to another, and their breakdown
into energy.

*Inclusions: functions of metabolism, basal metabolic
rate, metabolism of carbohydrate, protein and fat,
catabolism, anabolism, energy production in the body;
increase or decrease in metabolic rate*

*Exclusions: assimilation functions (b520); weight
maintenance functions (b530); water, mineral and
electrolyte balance functions (b545); thermoregulatory
functions (b550); endocrine glands functions (b555)*

b 545   **Water, mineral and electrolyte balance functions**
Functions of the regulation of water, mineral and
electrolytes in the body.

*Inclusions: functions of water balance, balance of
minerals such as calcium, zinc and iron, and balance of
electrolytes such as sodium and potassium; impairments
such as in water retention, dehydration,
hypercalcaemia, hypocalcaemia, iron deficiency,
hypernatraemia, hyponatraemia, hyperkalaemia and
hypokalaemia*

*Exclusions: haematological system functions (b430);
general metabolic functions (b540); endocrine gland
functions (b555)*

b 550   **Thermoregulatory functions**
Functions of the regulation of body temperature.

*Inclusions: functions of maintenance of body
temperature; impairments such as hypothermia,
hyperthermia*

*Exclusions: general metabolic functions (b540);
endocrine gland functions (b555)*

b 555 **Endocrine gland functions**
Functions of production and regulation of hormonal levels in the body, including cyclical changes.

Inclusions: functions of hormonal balance; hyperpituitarism, hypopituitarism, hyperthyroidism, hypothyroidism, hyperadrenalism, hypoadrenalism, hyperparathyroidism, hypoparathyroidism, hypergonadism, hypogonadism

Exclusions: general metabolic functions (b540); water, mineral and electrolyte balance functions (b545); thermoregulatory functions (b550); sexual functions (b640); menstruation functions (b650)

b 559 **Functions related to metabolism and the endocrine system, other specified and unspecified**

b 598 **Functions of the digestive, metabolic and endocrine systems, other specified**

b 599 **Functions of the digestive, metabolic and endocrine systems, unspecified**

Chapter 6

Genitourinary and reproductive functions

This chapter is about the functions of urination and the reproductive functions, including sexual and procreative functions.

Urinary functions (b610–b639)

b610   **Urinary excretory functions**
Functions of filtration and collection of the urine.

Inclusions: functions of urinary filtration, collection of urine; impairments such as in renal insufficiency, anuria, oliguria, hydronephrosis, hypotonic urinary bladder and ureteric obstruction

Exclusion: urination functions (b620)

b620   **Urination functions**
Functions of discharge of urine from the urinary bladder.

Inclusions: functions of urination, frequency of urination, urinary continence; impairments such as in stress, urge, reflex, overflow, continuous incontinence, dribbling, automatic bladder, polyuria, urinary retention and urinary urgency

Exclusions: urinary excretory functions (b610); sensations associated with urinary functions (b630)

b 630   **Sensations associated with urinary functions**
Sensations arising from voiding and related urinary functions

Inclusions: sensations of incomplete voiding of urine, feeling of fullness of bladder

Exclusions: sensations of pain (b280); urination functions (b620)

b 639   Urinary functions, other specified and unspecified

Genital and reproductive functions (b640-b679)

b 640   **Sexual functions**
Mental and physical functions related to the sexual act, including the arousal, preparatory, orgasmic and resolution stages.

Inclusions: functions of the sexual arousal, preparatory, orgasmic and resolution phase: functions related to sexual interest, performance, penile erection, clitoral erection, vaginal lubrication, ejaculation, orgasm; impairments such as impotence, frigidity, vaginismus, premature ejaculation, priapism and delayed ejaculation

Exclusions: procreation functions (b660); sensations associated with genital and reproductive functions (b670)

Menstruation functions

Functions associated with the menstrual cycle, including regularity of menstruation and discharge of menstrual fluids.

Inclusions: functions of regularity and interval of menstruation, extent of menstrual bleeding, menarche, menopause; impairments such as primary and secondary amenorrhoea, menorrhagia, polymenorrhoea and retrograde menstruationpremenstrual tension

Exclusions: sexual functions (b640); procreation functions (b660); sensations associated with genital and reproductive functions (b670); sensation of pain (b280)

 Procreation functions

Functions associated with fertility, pregnancy, childbirth and lactation.

Inclusions: functions of male fertility and female fertility, pregnancy and childbirth, and lactation; impairments such as azoospermia, oligozoospermia, agalactorrhoea, galactorrhoea, alactationand such as in subfertility, sterility, , spontaneous abortions, ectopic pregnancy, miscarriage, small fetus, hydramnios and premature childbirth, and delayed childbirth

Exclusions: sexual functions (b640); menstruation functions (b650)

b670 **Sensations associated with genital and reproductive functions**
Sensations arising from sexual arousal, intercourse, menstruation, and related genital or reproductive functions.

Inclusions: sensations of dyspareunia, dysmenorrhoea, hot flushes during menopause and night sweats during menopause

Exclusions: sensation of pain (b280); sensations associated with urinary functions (b630); sexual functions (b640); menstruation functions (b650); procreation functions (b660)

b679 **Genital and reproductive functions, other specified and unspecified**

b698 **Genitourinary and reproductive functions, other specified**

b699 **Genitourinary and reproductive functions, unspecified**

Chapter 7

Neuromusculoskeletal and movement-related functions

This chapter is about the functions of movement and mobility, including functions of joints, bones, reflexes and muscles.

Functions of the joints and bones (b710-b729)

b710 **Mobility of joint functions**
Functions of the range and ease of movement of a joint.

Inclusions: functions of mobility of single or several joints, vertebral, shoulder, elbow, wrist, hip, knee, ankle, small joints of hands and feet; mobility of joints generalized; impairments such as in hypermobility of joints, frozen joints, frozen shoulder, arthritis

Exclusions: stability of joint functions (b715); control of voluntary movement functions (b760)

b715   **Stability of joint functions**
Functions of the maintenance of structural integrity of the joints.

Inclusions: functions of the stability of a single joint, several joints, and joints generalized; impairments such as in unstable shoulder joint, dislocation of a joint, dislocation of shoulder and hip

Exclusion: mobility of joint functions (b710)

b720   **Mobility of bone functions**
Functions of the range and ease of movement of the scapula, pelvis, carpal and tarsal bones.

Inclusions: impairments such as frozen scapula and frozen pelvis

Exclusion: mobility of joints functions (b710)

b729   **Functions of the joints and bones, other specified and unspecified**

Muscle functions (b730-b749)

b730 **Muscle power functions**
Functions related to the force generated by the contraction of a muscle or muscle groups.

Inclusions: functions associated with the power of specific muscles and muscle groups, muscles of one limb, one side of the body, the lower half of the body, all limbs, the trunk and the body as a whole; impairments such as weakness of small muscles in feet and hands, muscle paresis, muscle paralysis, monoplegia, hemiplegia, paraplegia, quadriplegia and akinetic mutism

Exclusions: functions of structures adjoining the eye (b215); muscle tone functions (b735); muscle endurance functions (b740)

b735 **Muscle tone functions**
Functions related to the tension present in the resting muscles and the resistance offered when trying to move the muscles passively.

Inclusions: functions associated with the tension of isolated muscles and muscle groups, muscles of one limb, one side of the body and the lower half of the body, muscles of all limbs, muscles of the trunk, and all muscles of the body; impairments such as hypotonia, hypertonia and muscle spasticity

Exclusions: muscle power functions (b730); muscle endurance functions (b740)

b 740   **Muscle endurance functions**
Functions related to sustaining muscle contraction for
the required period of time.

*Inclusions: functions associated with sustaining muscle
contraction for isolated muscles and muscle groups, and
all muscles of the body; impairments such as in
myasthenia gravis*

*Exclusions: exercise tolerance functions (b455); muscle
power functions (b730); muscle tone functions (b735)*

b 749   **Muscle functions, other specified and unspecified**

Movement functions (b750-b789)

b 750   **Motor reflex functions**
Functions of involuntary contraction of muscles
automatically induced by specific stimuli.

*Inclusions: functions of stretch motor reflex, automatic
local joint reflex, reflexes generated by noxious stimuli
and other exteroceptive stimuli; withdrawal reflex,
biceps reflex, radius reflex, quadriceps reflex, patellar
reflex, ankle reflex*

b755 **Involuntary movement reaction functions**

Functions of involuntary contractions of large muscles or the whole body induced by body position, balance and threatening stimuli.

Inclusions: functions of postural reactions, righting reactions, body adjustment reactions, balance reactions, supporting reactions, defensive reactions

Exclusion: motor reflex functions (b750)

b760 **Control of voluntary movement functions**

Functions associated with control over and coordination of voluntary movements.

Inclusions: functions of control of simple voluntary movements and of complex voluntary movements, coordination of voluntary movements, supportive functions of arm or leg, right left motor coordination, eye hand coordination, eye foot coordination; impairments such as control and coordination problems, e.g. dysdiadochokinesia

Exclusions: muscle power functions (b730); involuntary movement functions (b765); gait pattern functions (b770)

b765 **Involuntary movement functions**
Functions of unintentional, non- or semi-purposive
involuntary contractions of a muscle or group of
muscles.

*Inclusions: involuntary contractions of muscles;
impairments such as tremors, tics, mannerisms,
stereotypies, motor perseveration, chorea, athetosis,
vocal tics, dystonic movements and dyskinesia*

*Exclusions: control of voluntary movement functions
(b760); gait pattern functions (b770)*

b770 **Gait pattern functions**
Functions of movement patterns associated with
walking, running or other whole body movements.

*Inclusions: walking patterns and running patterns;
impairments such as spastic gait, hemiplegic gait,
paraplegic gait, asymmetric gait, limping and stiff gait
pattern*

*Exclusions: muscle power functions (b730); muscle tone
functions (b735); control of voluntary movement
functions (b760); involuntary movement functions
(b765)*

b 780 **Sensations related to muscles and movement functions**

Sensations associated with the muscles or muscle groups of the body and their movement.

Inclusions: sensations of muscle stiffness and tightness of muscles, muscle spasm or constriction, and heaviness of muscles

Exclusion: sensation of pain (b280)

b 789 **Movement functions, other specified and unspecified**

b 798 **Neuromusculoskeletal and movement-related functions, other specified**

b 799 **Neuromusculoskeletal and movement-related functions, unspecified**

Chapter 8
Functions of the skin and related structures

This chapter is about the functions of skin, nails and hair.

Functions of the skin (b810-b849)

b810 **Protective functions of the skin**
Functions of the skin for protecting the body from physical, chemical and biological threats.

Inclusions: functions of protecting against the sun and other radiation, photosensitivity, pigmentation, quality of skin; insulating function of skin, callus formation, hardening; impairments such as broken skin, ulcers, bedsores and thinning of skin

Exclusions: repair functions of the skin (b820); other functions of the skin (b830)

b820 **Repair functions of the skin**
Functions of the skin for repairing breaks and other damage to the skin.

Inclusions: functions of scab formation, healing, scarring; bruising and keloid formation

Exclusions: protective functions of the skin (b810); other functions of the skin (b830)

b830 **Other functions of the skin**
Functions of the skin other than protection and repair, such as cooling and sweat secretion.

Inclusions: functions of sweating, glandular functions of the skin and resulting body odour

Exclusions: protective functions of the skin (b810); repair functions of the skin (b820)

b840 **Sensation related to the skin**
Sensations related to the skin such as itching, burning sensation and tingling.

Inclusions: impairments such as pins and needles sensation and crawling sensation

Exclusion: sensation of pain (b280)

b849 **Functions of the skin, other specified and unspecified**

Functions of the hair and nails (b850-b869)

b850 **Functions of hair**
Functions of the hair, such as protection, coloration and appearance.

Inclusions: functions of growth of hair, pigmentation of hair, location of hair; impairments such as loss of hair or alopecia

b 860   **Functions of nails**
Functions of the nails, such as protection, scratching and appearance.

Inclusions: growth and pigmentation of nails, quality of nails

b 869   **Functions of the hair and nails, other specified and unspecified**

b 898   **Functions of the skin and related structures, other specified**

b 899   **Functions of the skin and related structures, unspecified**

BODY STRUCTURES

Definitions: ***Body structures*** *are anatomical parts of the*
                          body such as organs, limbs and their
                          components.

                          Impairments *are problems in body function*
                          or structure as a significant deviation or loss.

First qualifier

Generic qualifier with the negative scale used to indicate the
extent or magnitude of an impairment:

xxx.0	NO impairment	(none, absent, negligible,…)	0-4 %
xxx.1	MILD impairment	(slight, low,…)	5-24 %
xxx.2	MODERATE impairment	(medium, fair,…)	25-49 %
xxx.3	SEVERE impairment	(high, extreme, …)	50-95 %
xxx.4	COMPLETE impairment	(total,…)	96-100 %
xxx.8	not specified		
xxx.9	not applicable		

Broad ranges of percentages are provided for those cases in
which calibrated assessment instruments or other standards are
available to quantify the impairment in body structure. For
example, when "no impairment" or "complete impairment" in
body structure is coded, this scaling may have margin of error of
up to 5%. "Moderate impairment" is generally up to half of the
scale of total impairment. The percentages are to be calibrated in
different domains with reference to population standards as
percentiles. For this quantification to be used in a uniform
manner, assessment procedures need to be developed through
research.

Second qualifier

Used to indicate the nature of the change in the respective body structure:

0	no change in structure
1	total absence
2	partial absence
3	additional part
4	aberrant dimensions
5	discontinuity
6	deviating position
7	qualitative changes in structure, including accumulation of fluid
8	not specified
9	not applicable

Third qualifier (suggested)

To be developed to indicate localization

0	more than one region
1	right
2	left
3	both sides
4	front
5	back
6	proximal
7	distal
8	not specified
9	not applicable

For a further explanation of coding conventions in ICF, refer to Annex 2.

Chapter 1
Structures of the nervous system

Chapter 2
The eye, ear and related structures

Chapter 3
Structures involved in voice and speech

Chapter 4
Structures of the cardio-vascular, immunological and respiratory systems

Chapter 5

Structures related to the digestive, metabolic and endocrine systems

Chapter 6
Structures related to the genitourinary and reproductive systems

s610 Structure of urinary system

s620 Structure of pelvic floor

s630 Structure of reproductive system

s698 Structures related to the genitourinary and reproductive systems, other specified

s699 Structures related to the genitourinary and reproductive systems, unspecified

Chapter 7
Structures related to movement

Chapter 8
Skin and related structures

s810 Structure of areas of skin

s820 Structure of skin glands

s830 Structure of nails

s840 Structure of hair

s898 Skin and related structures, other specified

s899 Skin and related structures, unspecifed

ACTIVITIES AND PARTICIPATION

Definitions: ***Activity*** *is the execution of a task or action by an individual.*

Participation *is involvement in a life situation.*

Activity limitations *are difficulties an individual may have in executing activities.*

Participation restrictions *are problems an individual may experience in involvement in life situations.*

Qualifiers

The domains for the Activities and Participation component are given in a single list that covers the full range of life areas (from basic learning and watching to composite areas such as social tasks). This component can be used to denote activities (a) or participation (p) or both.

The two qualifiers for the Activities and Participation component are the *performance* qualifier and the *capacity* qualifier. The performance qualifier describes what an individual does in his or her current environment. Because the current environment brings in a societal context, performance as recorded by this qualifier can also be understood as "involvement in a life situation" or "the lived experience" of people in the actual context in which they live. This context includes the environmental factors – all aspects of the physical, social and attitudinal world, which can be coded using the Environmental Factors component.

The capacity qualifier describes an individual's ability to execute a task or an action. This qualifier identifies the highest probable level of functioning that a person may reach in a given domain at a given moment. Capacity is measured in a uniform or standard environment, and thus reflects the environmentally adjusted ability of the individual. The Environmental Factors component can be used to describe the features of this uniform or standard environment.

Both capacity and performance qualifiers can be used both with and without assistive devices or personal assistance, and in accordance with the following scale:

xxx.0 NO difficulty	(none, absent, negligible,…)	0-4 %
xxx.1 MILD difficulty	(slight, low,…)	5-24 %
xxx.2 MODERATE difficulty	(medium, fair,...)	25-49 %
xxx.3 SEVERE difficulty	(high, extreme, …)	50-95 %
xxx.4 COMPLETE difficulty	(total,…)	96-100 %
xxx.8 not specified		
xxx.9 not applicable		

Broad ranges of percentages are provided for those cases in which calibrated assessment instruments or other standards are available to quantify the performance problem or capacity limitation. For example, when no performance problem or a complete performance problem is coded, this scaling has a margin of error of up to 5%. A moderate performance problem is defined as up to half of the scale of a total performance problem. The percentages are to be calibrated in different domains with reference to population standards as percentiles. For this quantification to be used in a uniform manner, assessment procedures need to be developed through research.

For a further explanation of coding convention in ICF, refer to Annex 2.

Chapter 1
Learning and applying knowledge

This chapter is about learning, applying the knowledge that is learned, thinking, solving problems, and making decisions.

Purposeful sensory experiences (d110-d129)

d110   **Watching**
Using the sense of seeing intentionally to experience visual stimuli, such as watching a sporting event or children playing.

d115   **Listening**
Using the sense of hearing intentionally to experience auditory stimuli, such as listening to a radio, music or a lecture.

d120   **Other purposeful sensing**
Using the body's other basic senses intentionally to experience stimuli, such as touching and feeling textures, tasting sweets or smelling flowers.

d129   **Purposeful sensory experiences, other specified and unspecified**

Basic learning (d130-d159)

d130   **Copying**
Imitating or mimicking as a basic component of learning, such as copying a gesture, a sound or the letters of an alphabet.

d135   **Rehearsing**
Repeating a sequence of events or symbols as a basic component of learning, such as counting by tens or practising the recitation of a poem.

d140   **Learning to read**
Developing the competence to read written material (including Braille) with fluency and accuracy, such as recognizing characters and alphabets, sounding out words with correct pronunciation, and understanding words and phrases.

d145   **Learning to write**
Developing the competence to produce symbols that represent sounds, words or phrases in order to convey meaning (including Braille writing), such as spelling effectively and using correct grammar.

d150   **Learning to calculate**
Developing the competence to manipulate numbers and perform simple and complex mathematical operations, such as using mathematical signs for addition and subtraction and applying the correct mathematical operation to a problem.

d155   **Acquiring skills**
Developing basic and complex competencies in integrated sets of actions or tasks so as to initiate and follow through with the acquisition of a skill, such as manipulating tools or playing games like chess.

Inclusions: acquiring basic and complex skills

d159   **Basic learning, other specified and unspecified**

Applying knowledge (d160-d179)

d160   **Focusing attention**
Intentionally focusing on specific stimuli, such as by filtering out distracting noises.

d163   **Thinking**
Formulating and manipulating ideas, concepts, and images, whether goal-oriented or not, either alone or with others, such as creating fiction, proving a theorem, playing with ideas, brainstorming, meditating, pondering, speculating, or reflecting.

Exclusions: solving problems (d175); making decisions (d177)

d166   **Reading**
Performing activities involved in the comprehension and interpretation of written language (e.g. books, instructions or newspapers in text or Braille), for the purpose of obtaining general knowledge or specific information.

Exclusion: learning to read (d140)

d 170   **Writing**
Using or producing symbols or language to convey information, such as producing a written record of events or ideas or drafting a letter.

Exclusion: learning to write (d145)

d 172   **Calculating**
Performing computations by applying mathematical principles to solve problems that are described in words and producing or displaying the results, such as computing the sum of three numbers or finding the result of dividing one number by another.

Exclusion: learning to calculate (d150)

d 175   **Solving problems**
Finding solutions to questions or situations by identifying and analysing issues, developing options and solutions, evaluating potential effects of solutions, and executing a chosen solution, such as in resolving a dispute between two people.

Inclusions: solving simple and complex problems

Exclusions: thinking (d163); making decisions (d177)

d 177   **Making decisions**
Making a choice among options, implementing the choice, and evaluating the effects of the choice, such as selecting and purchasing a specific item, or deciding to undertake and undertaking one task from among several tasks that need to be done.

Exclusions: thinking (d163); solving problems (d175)

d 179   Applying knowledge, other specified and unspecified

d 198   Learning and applying knowledge, other specified

d 199   Learning and applying knowledge, unspecified

Chapter 2

General tasks and demands

This chapter is about general aspects of carrying out single or multiple tasks, organizing routines and handling stress. These items can be used in conjunction with more specific tasks or actions to identify the underlying features of the execution of tasks under different circumstances.

d210   **Undertaking a single task**

Carrying out simple or complex and coordinated actions related to the mental and physical components of a single task, such as initiating a task, organizing time, space and materials for a task, pacing task performance, and carrying out, completing, and sustaining a task.

Inclusions: undertaking a simple or complex task; undertaking a single task independently or in a group

Exclusions: acquiring skills (d155); solving problems (d175); making decisions (d177); undertaking multiple tasks (d220)

d 220 **Undertaking multiple tasks**
Carrying out simple or complex and coordinated
actions as components of multiple, integrated and
complex tasks in sequence or simultaneously.

*Inclusions: undertaking multiple tasks; completing
multiple tasks; undertaking multiple tasks
independently and in a group*

*Exclusions: acquiring skills (d155); solving problems
(d175); making decisions (d177); undertaking a single
task (d210)*

d 230 **Carrying out daily routine**
Carrying out simple or complex and coordinated
actions in order to plan, manage and complete the
requirements of day-to-day procedures or duties, such
as budgeting time and making plans for separate
activities throughout the day.

*Inclusions: managing and completing the daily routine;
managing one's own activity level*

Exclusion: undertaking multiple tasks (d220)

d 240 **Handling stress and other psychological demands**
Carrying out simple or complex and coordinated
actions to manage and control the psychological
demands required to carry out tasks demanding
significant responsibilities and involving stress,
distraction, or crises, such as driving a vehicle during
heavy traffic or taking care of many children.

*Inclusions: handling responsibilities; handling stress
and crisis*

d 298   General tasks and demands, other specified

d 299   General tasks and demands, unspecified

Chapter 3
Communication

This chapter is about general and specific features of communicating by language, signs and symbols, including receiving and producing messages, carrying on conversations, and using communication devices and techniques.

Communicating - receiving (d310-d329)

d310   **Communicating with - receiving - spoken messages**
Comprehending literal and implied meanings of messages in spoken language, such as understanding that a statement asserts a fact or is an idiomatic expression.

d315   **Communicating with - receiving - nonverbal messages**
Comprehending the literal and implied meanings of messages conveyed by gestures, symbols and drawings, such as realizing that a child is tired when she rubs her eyes or that a warning bell means that there is a fire.

Inclusions: communicating with - receiving - body gestures, general signs and symbols, drawings and photographs

d320   **Communicating with - receiving - formal sign language messages**
Receiving and comprehending messages in formal sign language with literal and implied meaning.

d325　**Communicating with - receiving - written messages**
Comprehending the literal and implied meanings of
messages that are conveyed through written language
(including Braille), such as following political events in
the daily newspaper or understanding the intent of
religious scripture.

d329　Communicating - receiving, other specified and
unspecified

Communicating - producing (d330-d349)

d330　Speaking
Producing words, phrases and longer passages in
spoken messages with literal and implied meaning,
such as expressing a fact or telling a story in oral
language.

d335　Producing nonverbal messages
Using gestures, symbols and drawings to convey
messages, such as shaking one's head to indicate
disagreement or drawing a picture or diagram to
convey a fact or complex idea.

*Inclusions: producing body gestures, signs, symbols,
drawings and photographs*

d340　Producing messages in formal sign language
Conveying, with formal sign language, literal and
implied meaning.

d345 **Writing messages**
Producing the literal and implied meanings of
messages that are conveyed through written language,
such as writing a letter to a friend.

d349 Communication - producing, other specified and
unspecified

Conversation and use of communication devices and techniques (d350-d369)

d350 Conversation
Starting, sustaining and ending an interchange of
thoughts and ideas, carried out by means of spoken,
written, sign or other forms of language, with one or
more people one knows or who are strangers, in
formal or casual settings.

*Inclusions: starting, sustaining and ending a
conversation; conversing with one or many people*

d355 Discussion
Starting, sustaining and ending an examination of a
matter, with arguments for or against, or debate
carried out by means of spoken, written, sign or other
forms of language, with one or more people one knows
or who are strangers, in formal or casual settings.

Inclusion: discussion with one person or many people

d360 **Using communication devices and techniques**
Using devices, techniques and other means for the purposes of communicating, such as calling a friend on the telephone.

Inclusions: using telecommunication devices, using writing machines and communication techniques

d369 **Conversation and use of communication devices and techniques, other specified and unspecified**

d398 **Communication, other specified**

d399 **Communication, unspecified**

Chapter 4

Mobility

This chapter is about moving by changing body position or location or by transferring from one place to another, by carrying, moving or manipulating objects, by walking, running or climbing, and by using various forms of transportation.

Changing and maintaining body position (d410-d429)

d410   **Changing basic body position**
Getting into and out of a body position and moving from one location to another, such as getting up out of a chair to lie down on a bed, and getting into and out of positions of kneeling or squatting.

Inclusions: changing body position from lying down, from squatting or kneeling, from sitting or standing, bending and shifting the body's centre of gravity

Exclusion: transferring oneself (d420)

d415   **Maintaining a body position**
Staying in the same body position as required, such as remaining seated or remaining standing for work or school.

Inclusions: maintaining a lying, squatting, kneeling, sitting and standing position

d 420 **Transferring oneself**
Moving from one surface to another, such as sliding along a bench or moving from a bed to a chair, without changing body position.

Inclusions: transferring oneself while sitting or lying

Exclusion: changing basic body position (d410)

d 429 **Changing and maintaining body position, other specified and unspecified**

Carrying, moving and handling objects (d430-d449)

d 430 **Lifting and carrying objects**
Raising up an object or taking something from one place to another, such as when lifting a cup or carrying a child from one room to another.

Inclusions: lifting, carrying in the hands or arms, or on shoulders, hip, back or head; putting down

d 435 **Moving objects with lower extremities**
Performing coordinated actions aimed at moving an object by using the legs and feet, such as kicking a ball or pushing pedals on a bicycle.

Inclusions: pushing with lower extremities; kicking

d 440 Fine hand use

Performing the coordinated actions of handling objects, picking up, manipulating and releasing them using one's hand, fingers and thumb, such as required to lift coins off a table or turn a dial or knob.

Inclusions: picking up, grasping, manipulating and releasing

Exclusion: lifting and carrying objects (d430)

d 445 Hand and arm use

Performing the coordinated actions required to move objects or to manipulate them by using hands and arms, such as when turning door handles or throwing or catching an object.

Inclusions: pulling or pushing objects; reaching; turning or twisting the hands or arms; throwing; catching

Exclusion: fine hand use (d440)

d 449 Carrying, moving and handling objects, other specified and unspecified

Walking and moving (d450-d469)

d 450   Walking

Moving along a surface on foot, step by step, so that one foot is always on the ground, such as when strolling, sauntering, walking forwards, backwards, or sideways.

Inclusions: walking short or long distances; walking on different surfaces; walking around obstacles

Exclusions: transferring oneself (d420); moving around (d455)

d 455   Moving around

Moving the whole body from one place to another by means other than walking, such as climbing over a rock or running down a street, skipping, scampering, jumping, somersaulting or running around obstacles.

Inclusions: crawling, climbing, running, jogging, jumping, and swimming

Exclusions: transferring oneself (d420); walking (d450)

d 460 **Moving around in different locations**
Walking and moving around in various places and
situations, such as walking between rooms in a house,
within a building, or down the street of a town.

*Inclusions: moving around within the home, crawling or
climbing within the home; walking or moving within
buildings other than the home, and outside the home
and other buildings*

d 465 **Moving around using equipment**
Moving the whole body from place to place, on any
surface or space, by using specific devices designed to
facilitate moving or create other ways of moving
around, such as with skates, skis, or scuba equipment,
or moving down the street in a wheelchair or a walker.

*Exclusions: transferring oneself (d420); walking (d450);
moving around (d455); using transportation (d470);
driving (d475)*

d 469 **Walking and moving, other specified and
unspecified**

Moving around using transportation (d470-d489)

d470 **Using transportation**

Using transportation to move around as a passenger, such as being driven in a car or on a bus, rickshaw, jitney, animal-powered vehicle, or private or public taxi, bus, train, tram, subway, boat or aircraft.

Inclusions: using human-powered transportation; using private motorized or public transportation

Exclusions: moving around using equipment (d465); driving (d475)

d475 **Driving**

Being in control of and moving a vehicle or the animal that draws it, travelling under one's own direction or having at one's disposal any form of transportation, such as a car, bicycle, boat or animal-powered vehicle.

Inclusions: driving human-powered transportation, motorized vehicles, animal-powered vehicles

Exclusions: moving around using equipment (d465); using transportation (d470)

d480 **Riding animals for transportation**

travelling on the back of an animal, such as a horse, ox, camel or elephant

Exclusions: driving (d475); recreation and leisure (d920)

d 489 Moving around using transportation, other specified and unspecified

d 498 Mobility, other specified

d 499 Mobility, unspecified

Chapter 5
Self-care

This chapter is about caring for oneself, washing and drying oneself, caring for one's body and body parts, dressing, eating and drinking, and looking after one's health.

d510   **Washing oneself**

Washing and drying one's whole body, or body parts, using water and appropriate cleaning and drying materials or methods, such as bathing, showering, washing hands and feet, face and hair, and drying with a towel.

Inclusions: washing body parts, the whole body; and drying oneself

Exclusions: caring for body parts (d520); toileting (d530)

d520   **Caring for body parts**

Looking afer those parts of the body, such as skin, face, teeth, scalp, nails and genitals, that require more than washing and drying.

Inclusions: caring for skin, teeth, hair, finger and toe nails

Exclusions: washing oneself (d510); toileting (d530)

d530 **Toileting**
Planning and carrying out the elimination of human
waste (menstruation, urination and defecation), and
cleaning oneself afterwards.

*Inclusions: regulating urination, defecation and
menstrual care*

*Exclusions: washing oneself (d510); caring for body
parts (d520)*

d540 **Dressing**
Carrying out the coordinated actions and tasks of
putting on and taking off clothes and footwear in
sequence and in keeping with climatic and social
conditions, such as by putting on, adjusting and
removing shirts, skirts, blouses, pants, undergarments,
saris, kimono, tights, hats, gloves, coats, shoes, boots,
sandals and slippers.

*Inclusions: putting on or taking off clothes and footwear
and choosing appropriate clothing*

d550 **Eating**
Carrying out the coordinated tasks and actions of
eating food that has been served, bringing it to the
mouth and consuming it in culturally acceptable ways,
cutting or breaking food into pieces, opening bottles
and cans, using eating implements, having meals,
feasting or dining.

Exclusion: drinking (d560)

d560   **Drinking**
Taking hold of a drink, bringing it to the mouth, and
consuming the drink in culturally acceptable ways,
mixing, stirring and pouring liquids for drinking,
opening bottles and cans, drinking through a straw or
drinking running water such as from a tap or a spring;
feeding from the breast.

Exclusion: eating (d550)

d570   **Looking after one's health**
Ensuring physical comfort, health and physical and
mental well-being, such as by maintaining a balanced
diet, and an appropriate level of physical activity,
keeping warm or cool, avoiding harms to health,
following safe sex practices, including using condoms,
getting immunizations and regular physical
examinations.

*Inclusions: ensuring one's physical comfort; managing
diet and fitness; maintaining one's health*

d598   **Self-care, other specified**

d599   **Self-care, unspecified**

Chapter 6

Domestic life

This chapter is about carrying out domestic and everyday actions and tasks. Areas of domestic life include acquiring a place to live, food, clothing and other necessities, household cleaning and repairing, caring for personal and other household objects, and assisting others.

Acquisition of necessities (d610-d629)

d610   **Acquiring a place to live**
Buying, renting, furnishing and arranging a house, apartment or other dwelling.

Inclusions: buying or renting a place to live and furnishing a place to live

Exclusions: acquisition of goods and services (d620); caring for household objects (d650)

d620   **Acquisition of goods and services**
Selecting, procuring and transporting all goods and services required for daily living, such as selecting, procuring, transporting and storing food, drink, clothing, cleaning materials, fuel, household items, utensils, cooking ware, domestic appliance and tools; procuring utilities and other household services.

Inclusions: shopping and gathering daily necessities

Exclusion: acquiring a place to live (d610)

d 629   Acquisition of necessities, other specified and unspecified

Household tasks (d630-d649)

d 630   Preparing meals

Planning, organizing, cooking and serving simple and complex meals for oneself and others, such as by making a menu, selecting edible food and drink, getting together ingredients for preparing meals, cooking with heat and preparing cold foods and drinks, and serving the food.

Inclusions: preparing simple and complex meals

Exclusions: eating (d550); drinking (d560); acquisition of goods and services (d620); doing housework (d640); caring for household objects (d650); caring for others (d660)

d640   Doing housework

Managing a household by cleaning the house, washing clothes, using household appliances, storing food and disposing of garbage, such as by sweeping, mopping, washing counters, walls and other surfaces; collecting and disposing of household garbage; tidying rooms, closets and drawers; collecting, washing, drying, folding and ironing clothes; cleaning footwear; using brooms, brushes and vacuum cleaners; using washing machines, driers and irons.

Inclusions: washing and drying clothes and garments; cleaning cooking area and utensils; cleaning living area; using household appliances, storing daily necessities and disposing of garbage

Exclusions: acquiring a place to live (d610); acquisition of goods and services (d620); preparing meals (d630); caring for household objects (d650); caring for others (d660)

d649   Household tasks, other specified and unspecified

Caring for household objects and assisting others (d650-d669)

d650 **Caring for household objects**
Maintaining and repairing household and other personal objects, including house and contents, clothes, vehicles and assistive devices, and caring for plants and animals, such as painting or wallpapering rooms, fixing furniture, repairing plumbing, ensuring the proper working order of vehicles, watering plants, grooming and feeding pets and domestic animals.

Inclusions: making and repairing clothes; maintaining dwelling, furnishings and domestic appliances; maintaining vehicles; maintaining assistive devices; taking care of plants (indoor and outdoor) and animals

Exclusions: acquiring a place to live (d610); acquisition of goods and services (d620); doing housework (d640); caring for others (d660); remunerative employment (d850)

d660 **Assisting others**
Assisting household members and others with their learning, communicating, self-care, movement, within the house or outside; being concerned about the well-being of household members and others.

Inclusions: assisting others with self-care, movement, communication, interpersonal relations, nutrition and health maintenance

Exclusion: remunerative employment (d850)

d 669   Caring for household objects and assisting others, other specified and unspecified

d 698   Domestic life, other specified

d 699   Domestic life, unspecified

Chapter 7

Interpersonal interactions and relationships

This chapter is about carrying out the actions and tasks required for basic and complex interactions with people (strangers, friends, relatives, family members and lovers) in a contextually and socially appropriate manner.

General interpersonal interactions (d710-d729)

d710 **Basic interpersonal interactions**
Interacting with people in a contextually and socially appropriate manner, such as by showing consideration and esteem when appropriate, or responding to the feelings of others.

Inclusions: showing respect, warmth, appreciation, and tolerance in relationships; responding to criticism and social cues in relationships; and using appropriate physical contact in relationships

d720   **Complex interpersonal interactions**
Maintaining and managing interactions with other
people, in a contextually and socially appropriate
manner, such as by regulating emotions and impulses,
controlling verbal and physical aggression, acting
independently in social interactions, and acting in
accordance with social rules and conventions.

*Inclusions: forming and terminating relationships;
regulating behaviours within interactions; interacting
according to social rules; and maintaining social space*

d729   **General interpersonal interactions, other specified
and unspecified**

Particular interpersonal relationships (d730-d779)

d730   **Relating with strangers**
Engaging in temporary contacts and links with
strangers for specific purposes, such as when asking
for directions or making a purchase.

d740   **Formal relationships**
Creating and maintaining specific relationships in
formal settings, such as with employers, professionals
or service providers.

*Inclusions: relating with persons in authority, with
subordinates and with equals*

d 750   **Informal social relationships**
Entering into relationships with others, such as casual
relationships with people living in the same
community or residence, or with co-workers, students,
playmates or people with similar backgrounds or
professions.

*Inclusions: informal relationships with friends,
neighbours, acquaintances, co-inhabitants and peers*

d 760   **Family relationships**
Creating and maintaining kinship relationships, such
as with members of the nuclear family, extended
family, foster and adopted family and step-
relationships, more distant relationships such as
second cousins, or legal guardians.

*Inclusions: parent-child and child-parent relationships,
sibling and extended family relationships*

d 770   **Intimate relationships**
Creating and maintaining close or romantic
relationships between individuals, such as husband
and wife, lovers or sexual partners.

Inclusions: romantic, spousal and sexual relationships

d 779   **Particular interpersonal relationships, other
specified and unspecified**

d 798   **Interpersonal interactions and relationships, other
specified**

d 799   **Interpersonal interactions and relationships,
unspecified**

Chapter 8
Major life areas

This chapter is about carrying out the tasks and actions required to engage in education, work and employment and to conduct economic transactions.

Education (d810-d839)

d810   **Informal education**
Learning at home or in some other non-institutional setting, such as learning crafts and other skills from parents or family members, or home schooling.

d815   **Preschool education**
Learning at an initial level of organized instruction, designed primarily to introduce a child to the school-type environment and prepare it for compulsory education, such as by acquiring skills in a day-care or similar setting as preparation for advancement to school.

d820   **School education**
Gaining admission to school, Education, engaging in all school-related responsibilities and privileges, and learning the course material, subjects and other curriculum requirements in a primary or secondary education programme, including attending school regularly, working cooperatively with other students, taking direction from teachers, organizing, studying and completing assigned tasks and projects, and advancing to other stages of education.

d 825 **Vocational training**

Engaging in all activities of a vocational programme and learning the curriculum material in preparation for employment in a trade, job or profession.

d 830 **Higher education**

Engaging in the activities of advanced educational programmes in universities, colleges and professional schools and learning all aspects of the curriculum required for degrees, diplomas, certificates and other accreditations, such as completing a university bachelor's or master's course of study, medical school or other professional school.

d 839 **Education, other specified and unspecified**

Work and employment (d840–d859)

d 840 **Apprenticeship (work preparation)**

Engaging in programmes related to preparation for employment, such as performing the tasks required of an apprenticeship, internship, articling and in-service training.

Exclusion: vocational training (d825)

d 845 **Acquiring, keeping and terminating a job**
Seeking, finding and choosing employment, being
hired and accepting employment, maintaining and
advancing through a job, trade, occupation or
profession, and leaving a job in an appropriate
manner.

*Inclusions: seeking employment; preparing a resume or
curriculum vitae; contacting employers and preparing
interviews; maintaining a job; monitoring one's own
work performance; giving notice; and terminating a job*

d 850 **Remunerative employment**
Engaging in all aspects of work, as an occupation,
trade, profession or other form of employment, for
payment, as an employee, full or part time, or self-
employed, such as seeking employment and getting a
job, doing the required tasks of the job, attending work
on time as required, supervising other workers or
being supervised, and performing required tasks alone
or in groups.

*Inclusions: self-employment, part-time and full-time
employment*

d 855 **Non-remunerative employment**

Engaging in all aspects of work in which pay is not provided, full-time or part-time, including organized work activities, doing the required tasks of the job, attending work on time as required, supervising other workers or being supervised, and performing required tasks alone or in groups, such as volunteer work, charity work, working for a community or religious group without remuneration, working around the home without remuneration.

Exclusion: Chapter 6 Domestic Life

d 859 **Work and employment, other specified and unspecified**

Economic life (d860-d879)

d 860 **Basic economic transactions**

Engaging in any form of simple economic transaction, such as using money to purchase food or bartering, exchanging goods or services; or saving money.

d 865 **Complex economic transactions**

Engaging in any form of complex economic transaction that involves the exchange of capital or property, and the creation of profit or economic value, such as buying a business, factory, or equipment, maintaining a bank account, or trading in commodities.

d870 **Economic self-sufficiency**
Having command over economic resources, from
private or public sources, in order to ensure economic
security for present and future needs.

*Inclusions: personal economic resources and public
economic entitlements*

d879 **Economic life, other specified and unspecified**

d898 **Major life areas, other specified**

d899 **Major life areas, unspecified**

Chapter 9

Community, social and civic life

This chapter is about the actions and tasks required to engage in organized social life outside the family, in community, social and civic areas of life.

d910   **Community life**

Engaging in all aspects of community social life, such as engaging in charitable organizations, service clubs or professional social organizations.

Inclusions: informal and formal associations; ceremonies

Exclusions: non-remunerative employment (d855); recreation and leisure (d920); religion and spirituality (d930); political life and citizenship (d950)

d 920   **Recreation and leisure**
Engaging in any form of play, recreational or leisure
activity, such as informal or organized play and sports,
programmes of physical fitness, relaxation,
amusement or diversion, going to art galleries,
museums, cinemas or theatres; engaging in crafts or
hobbies, reading for enjoyment, playing musical
instruments; sightseeing, tourism and travelling for
pleasure.

*Inclusions: play, sports, arts and culture, crafts, hobbies
and socializing*

*Exclusions: riding animals for transportation (d480);
remunerative and non-remunerative work (d850 and
d855); religion and spirituality (d930); political life and
citizenship (d950)*

d 930   **Religion and spirituality**
Engaging in religious or spiritual activities,
organizations and practices for self-fulfilment, finding
meaning, religious or spiritual value and establishing
connection with a divine power, such as is involved in
attending a church, temple, mosque or synagogue,
praying or chanting for a religious purpose, and
spiritual contemplation.

Inclusions: organized religion and spirituality

d940 **Human rights**
Enjoying all nationally and internationally recognized rights that are accorded to people by virtue of their humanity alone, such as human rights as recognized by the United Nations Universal Declaration of Human Rights (1948) and the United Nations Standard Rules for the Equalization of Opportunities for Persons with Disabilities (1993); the right to self-determination or autonomy; and the right to control over one's destiny.

Exclusion: political life and citizenship (d950)

d950 **Political life and citizenship**
Engaging in the social, political and governmental life of a citizen, having legal status as a citizen and enjoying the rights, protections, privileges and duties associated with that role, such as the right to vote and run for political office, to form political associations; enjoying the rights and freedoms associated with citizenship (e.g. the rights of freedom of speech, association, religion, protection against unreasonable search and seizure, the right to counsel, to a trial and other legal rights and protection against discrimination); having legal standing as a citizen.

Exclusion: human rights (d940)

d998 Community, social and civic life, other specified

d999 Community, social and civic life, unspecified

ENVIRONMENTAL FACTORS

Definition: *Environmental factors make up the physical, social and attitudinal environment in which people live and conduct their lives.*

Coding environmental factors

Environmental Factors is a component of Part 2 (Contextual factors) of the classification. These factors must be considered for each component of functioning and coded accordingly (see Annex 2).

Environmental factors are to be coded from the perspective of the person whose situation is being described. For example, kerb cuts without textured paving may be coded as a facilitator for a wheelchair user but as a barrier for a blind person.

The first qualifier indicates the extent to which a factor is a facilitator or a barrier. There are several reasons why an environmental factor may be a facilitator or a barrier, and to what extent. For facilitators, the coder should keep in mind issues such as the accessibility of a resource, and whether access is dependable or variable, of good or poor quality, and so on. In the case of barriers, it might be relevant how often a factor hinders the person, whether the hindrance is great or small, or avoidable or not. It should also be kept in mind that an environmental factor can be a barrier either because of its presence (for example, negative attitudes towards people with disabilities) or its absence (for example, the unavailability of a needed service). The effects that environmental factors have on the lives of people with health conditions are varied and complex, and it is hoped that future research will lead to better understanding of this interaction and, possibly, show the usefulness of a second qualifier for these factors.

In some instances, a diverse collection of environmental factors is summarized with a single term, such as poverty, development, rural or urban setting or social capital. These summary terms are not themselves found in the classification. Rather, the coder should separate the constituent factors and code these. Once again, further research is required to determine whether there are clear and consistent sets of environmental factors that make up each of these summary terms.

First qualifier
The following is the negative and positive scale for the extent to which an environmental factor acts as a barrier or a facilitator. A point or separator alone denotes a barrier, and the + sign denotes a facilitator, as indicated below:

xxx.0 NO barrier	(none, absent, negligible,...)	0-4%
xxx.1 MILD barrier	(slight, low,...)	5-24%
xxx.2 MODERATE barrier	(medium, fair,...)	25-49%
xxx.3 SEVERE barrier	(high, extreme, ...)	50-95%
xxx.4 COMPLETE barrier	(total,...)	96-100%

xxx+0 NO facilitator	(none, absent, negligible,...)	0-4%
xxx+1 MILD facilitator	(slight, low,...)	5-24%
xxx+2 MODERATE facilitator	(medium, fair,...)	25-49%
xxx+3 SUBSTANTIAL facilitator	(high, extreme, ...)	50-95%
xxx+4 COMPLETE facilitator	(total,...)	96-100%

xxx.8 barrier, not specified
xxx+8 facilitator, not specified
xxx.9 not applicable

Broad ranges of percentages are provided for those cases in which calibrated assessment instruments or other standards are available to quantify the extent of the barrier or facilitator in the environment. For example, when "no barrier" or a "complete barrier" is coded, this scaling has a margin of error of up to 5%. A "moderate barrier" is defined as up to half of the scale of a total barrier. The percentages are to be calibrated in different domains with reference to population standards as percentiles. For this quantification to be used in a uniform manner, assessment procedures have to be developed through research.

Second qualifier: To be developed.

Chapter 1

Products and technology

This chapter is about the natural or human-made products or systems of products, equipment and technology in an individual's immediate environment that are gathered, created, produced or manufactured. The ISO 9999 classification of technical aids defines these as "any product, instrument, equipment or technical system used by a disabled person, especially produced or generally available, preventing, compensating, monitoring, relieving or neutralizing" disability. It is recognized that any product or technology can be assistive. (See ISO 9999: Technical aids for disabled persons - Classification (second version); ISO/TC 173/SC 2; ISO/DIS 9999 (rev.).) For the purposes of this classification of environmental factors, however, assistive products and technology are defined more narrowly as any product, instrument, equipment or technology adapted or specially designed for improving the functioning of a disabled person.

 Products or substances for personal consumption
Any natural or human-made object or substance gathered, processed or manufactured for ingestion.

Inclusion: food and drugs

e115   **Products and technology for personal use in daily living**
Equipment, products and technologies used by people in daily activities, including those adapted or specially designed, located in, on or near the person using them.

Inclusions: general and assistive products and technology for personal use

e120   **Products and technology for personal indoor and outdoor mobility and transportation**
Equipment, products and technologies used by people in activities of moving inside and outside buildings, including those adapted or specially designed, located in, on or near the person using them.

Inclusions: general and assistive products and technology for personal indoor and outdoor mobility and transportation

e125   **Products and technology for communication**
Equipment, products and technologies used by people in activities of sending and receiving information, including those adapted or specially designed, located in, on or near the person using them.

Inclusions: general and assistive products and technology for communication

e130 **Products and technology for education**
Equipment, products, processes, methods and
technology used for acquisition of knowledge,
expertise or skill, including those adapted or specially
designed.

*Inclusions: general and assistive products and
technology for education*

e135 **Products and technology for employment**
Equipment, products and technology used for
employment to facilitate work activities.

*Inclusions: general and assistive products and
technology for employment*

e140 **Products and technology for culture, recreation and
sport**
Equipment, products and technology used for the
conduct and enhancement of cultural, recreational and
sporting activities, including those adapted or specially
designed.

*Inclusions: general and assistive products and
technology for culture, recreation and sport*

e145   **Products and technology for the practice of religion and spirituality**
Products and technology, unique or mass-produced, that are given or take on a symbolic meaning in the context of the practice of religion or spirituality, including those adapted or specially designed.

Inclusions: general and assistive products and technology for the practice of religion and spirituality

e150   **Design, construction and building products and technology of buildings for public use**
Products and technology that constitute an individual's indoor and outdoor human-made environment that is planned, designed and constructed for public use, including those adapted or specially designed.

Inclusions: design, construction and building products and technology of entrances and exits, facilities and routing

e155   **Design, construction and building products and technology of buildings for private use**
Products and technology that constitute an individual's indoor and outdoor human-made environment that is planned, designed and constructed for private use, including those adapted or specially designed.

Inclusions: design, construction and building products and technology of entrances and exits, facilities and routing

e160   **Products and technology of land development**
Products and technology of land areas, as they affect
an individual's outdoor environment through the
implementation of land use policies, design, planning
and development of space, including those adapted or
specially designed.

*Inclusions: products and technology of land areas that
have been organized by the implementation of land use
policies, such as rural areas, suburban areas, urban
areas, parks, conservation areas and wildlife reserves*

e165   **Assets**
Products or objects of economic exchange such as
money, goods, property and other valuables that an
individual owns or of which he or she has rights of use.

*Inclusions: tangible and intangible products and goods,
financial assets*

e198   **Products and technology, other specified**

e199   **Products and technology, unspecified**

Chapter 2
Natural environment and human-made changes to environment

This chapter is about animate and inanimate elements of the natural or physical environment, and components of that environment that have been modified by people, as well as characteristics of human populations within that environment.

e210   **Physical geography**
Features of land forms and bodies of water.

Inclusions: features of geography included within orography (relief, quality and expanse of land and land forms, including altitude) and hydrography (bodies of water such as lakes, rivers, sea)

e215   **Population**
Groups of people living in a given environment who share the same pattern of environmental adaptation.

Inclusions: demographic change; population density

e220   **Flora and fauna**
Plants and animals.

Exclusions: domesticated animals (e350); population (e215)

e225   **Climate**
Meteorological features and events, such as the weather.

Inclusions: temperature, humidity, atmospheric pressure, precipitation, wind and seasonal variations

e230   **Natural events**
Geographic and atmospheric changes that cause disruption in an individual's physical environment, occurring regularly or irregularly, such as earthquakes and severe or violent weather conditions, e.g. tornadoes, hurricanes, typhoons, floods, forest fires and ice-storms.

e235   **Human-caused events**
Alterations or disturbances in the natural environment, caused by humans, that may result in the disruption of people's day-to-day lives, including events or conditions linked to conflict and wars, such as the displacement of people, destruction of social infrastructure, homes and lands, environmental disasters and land, water or air pollution (e.g. toxic spills).

e240   **Light**
Electromagnetic radiation by which things are made visible by either sunlight or artificial lighting (e.g. candles, oil or paraffin lamps, fires and electricity), and which may provide useful or distracting information about the world.

Inclusions: light intensity; light quality; colour contrasts

e 245   **Time-related changes**
Natural, regular or predictable temporal change.

Inclusions: day/night and lunar cycles

e 250   **Sound**
A phenomenon that is or may be heard, such as
banging, ringing, thumping, singing, whistling, yelling
or buzzing, in any volume, timbre or tone, and that
may provide useful or distracting information about
the world.

Inclusions: sound intensity; sound quality

e 255   **Vibration**
Regular or irregular to and fro motion of an object or
an individual caused by a physical disturbance, such as
shaking, quivering, quick jerky movements of things,
buildings or people caused by small or large
equipment, aircraft and explosions.

*Exclusion: natural events (e230), such as vibration or
shaking of the earth caused by earthquakes*

e 260   **Air quality**
Characteristics of the atmosphere (outside buildings)
or enclosed areas of air (inside buildings), and which
may provide useful or distracting information about
the world.

Inclusions: indoor and outdoor air quality

e 298   **Natural environment and human-made changes to
environment, other specified**

e 299   **Natural environment and human-made changes to
environment, unspecified**

Chapter 3
Support and relationships

This chapter is about people or animals that provide practical physical or emotional support, nurturing, protection, assistance and relationships to other persons, in their home, place of work, school or at play or in other aspects of their daily activities. The chapter does not encompass the attitudes of the person or people that are providing the support. The environmental factor being described is not the person or animal, but the amount of physical and emotional support the person or animal provides.

e310   **Immediate family**
Individuals related by birth, marriage or other relationship recognized by the culture as immediate family, such as spouses, partners, parents, siblings, children, foster parents, adoptive parents and grandparents.

Exclusions: extended family (e315); personal care providers and personal assistants (e340)

e315   **Extended family**
Individuals related through family or marriage or other relationships recognized by the culture as extended family, such as aunts, uncles, nephews and nieces.

Exclusion: immediate family (e310)

e320 **Friends**
Individuals who are close and ongoing participants in relationships characterized by trust and mutual support.

e325 **Acquaintances, peers, colleagues, neighbours and community members**
Individuals who are familiar to each other as acquaintances, peers, colleagues, neighbours, and community members, in situations of work, school, recreation, or other aspects of life, and who share demographic features such as age, gender, religious creed or ethnicity or pursue common interests.

Exclusions: associations and organizational services (e5550)

e330 **People in positions of authority**
Individuals who have decision-making responsibilities for others and who have socially defined influence or power based on their social, economic, cultural or religious roles in society, such as teachers, employers, supervisors, religious leaders, substitute decision-makers, guardians or trustees.

e335 **People in subordinate positions**
Individuals whose day-to-day life is influenced by people in positions of authority in work, school or other settings, such as students, workers and members of a religious group.

Exclusion: immediate family (e310)

e340 **Personal care providers and personal assistants**
Individuals who provide services as required to support individuals in their daily activities and maintenance of performance at work, education or other life situation, provided either through public or private funds, or else on a voluntary basis, such as providers of support for home-making and maintenance, personal assistants, transport assistants, paid help, nannies and others who function as primary caregivers.

Exclusions: immediate family (e310); extended family (e315); friends (e320); general social support services (e5750); health professionals (e355)

e345 **Strangers**
Individuals who are unfamiliar and unrelated, or those who have not yet established a relationship or association, including persons unknown to the individual but who are sharing a life situation with them, such as substitute teachers co-workers or care providers.

e350 **Domesticated animals**
Animals that provide physical, emotional, or psychological support, such as pets (dogs, cats, birds, fish, etc.) and animals for personal mobility and transportation.

Exclusions: animals (e2201); assets (e165)

e355 **Health professionals**
All service providers working within the context of the health system, such as doctors, nurses, physiotherapists, occupational therapists, speech therapists, audiologists, orthotist-prosthetists, medical social workers.

Exclusion: other professionals (e360)

e360 **Other professionals**
All service providers working outside the health system, including social workers, lawyers, teachers, architects, and designers.

Exclusion: health professionals (e355)

e398 Support and relationships, other specified

e399 Support and relationships, unspecified

Chapter 4

Attitudes

This chapter is about the attitudes that are the observable
consequences of customs, practices, ideologies, values, norms,
factual beliefs and religious beliefs. These attitudes influence
individual behaviour and social life at all levels, from
interpersonal relationships and community associations to
political, economic and legal structures; for example, individual
or societal attitudes about a person's trustworthiness and value as
a human being may motivate positive, honorific practices or
negative and discriminatory practices (e.g. stigmatizing,
stereotyping and marginalizing or neglect of the person).   The
attitudes classified are those of people external to the person
whose situation is being described. They are not those of the
person themselves. The individual attitudes are categorized
according to the kinds of relationships listed in Environmental
Factors Chapter 3. Values and beliefs are not coded separately
from attitudes as they are assumed to be the driving forces
behind the attitudes.

e410 **Individual attitudes of immediate family members**
General or specific opinions and beliefs of immediate
family members about the person or about other
matters (e.g. social, political and economic issues), that
influence individual behaviour and actions.

e415 **Individual attitudes of extended family members**
General or specific opinions and beliefs of extended
family members about the person or about other
matters (e.g. social, political and economic issues), that
influence individual behaviour and actions.

e420 **Individual attitudes of friends**
General or specific opinions and beliefs of friends
about the person or about other matters (e.g. social,
political and economic issues), that influence
individual behaviour and actions.

e425 **Individual attitudes of acquaintances, peers,
colleagues, neighbours and community members**
General or specific opinions and beliefs of
acquaintances, peers, colleagues, neighbours and
community members about the person or about other
matters (e.g. social, political and economic issues), that
influence individual behaviour and actions.

e430 **Individual attitudes of people in positions of
authority**
General or specific opinions and beliefs of people in
positions of authority about the person or about other
matters (e.g. social, political and economic issues), that
influence individual behaviour and actions.

e435 **Individual attitudes of people in subordinate
positions**
General or specific opinions and beliefs of people in
subordinate positions about the person or about other
matters (e.g. social, political and economic issues), that
influence individual behaviour and actions.

e440 **Individual attitudes of personal care providers and personal assistants**
General or specific opinions and beliefs of personal care providers and personal assistants about the person or about other matters (e.g. social, political and economic issues), that influence individual behaviour and actions.

e445 **Individual attitudes of strangers**
General or specific opinions and beliefs of strangers about the person or about other matters (e.g. social, political and economic issues), that influence individual behaviour and actions.

e450 **Individual attitudes of health professionals**
General or specific opinions and beliefs of health professionals about the person or about other matters (e.g. social, political and economic issues), that influence individual behaviour and actions.

e455 **Individual attitudes of other professionals**
General or specific opinions and beliefs of health-related and other professionals about the person or about other matters (e.g. social, political and economic issues), that influence individual behaviour and actions.

e 460 **Societal attitudes**
General or specific opinions and beliefs generally held
by people of a culture, society, subcultural or other
social group about other individuals or about other
social, political and economic issues, that influence
group or individual behaviour and actions.

e 465 **Social norms, practices and ideologies**
Customs, practices, rules and abstract systems of
values and normative beliefs (e.g. ideologies,
normative world views and moral philosophies) that
arise within social contexts and that affect or create
societal and individual practices and behaviours, such
as social norms of moral and religious behaviour or
etiquette; religious doctrine and resulting norms and
practices; norms governing rituals or social gatherings.

e 498 **Attitudes, other specified**

e 499 **Attitudes, unspecified**

Chapter 5
Services, systems and policies

This chapter is about:

1. *Services* that provide benefits, structured programmes and operations, in various sectors of society, designed to meet the needs of individuals. (Included in services are the people who provide them.) Services may be public, private or voluntary, and may be established at a local, community, regional, state, provincial, national or international level by individuals, associations, organizations, agencies or governments. The goods provided by these services may be general or adapted and specially designed.

2. *Systems* that are administrative control and organizational mechanisms, and are established by governments at the local, regional, national, and international levels, or by other recognized authorities. These systems are designed to organize, control and monitor services that provide benefits, structured programmes and operations in various sectors of society.

3. *Policies* constituted by rules, regulations, conventions and standards established by governments at the local, regional, national, and international levels, or by other recognized authorities. Policies govern and regulate the systems that organize, control and monitor services, structured programmes and operations in various sectors of society.

e510 **Services, systems and policies for the production of consumer goods**
Services, systems and policies that govern and provide for the production of objects and products consumed or used by people.

e515 **Architecture and construction services, systems and policies**
Services, systems and policies for the design and construction of buildings, public and private.

Exclusion: open space planning services, systems and policies (e520)

e520 **Open space planning services, systems and policies**
Services, systems and policies for the planning, design, development and maintenance of public lands, (e.g. parks, forests, shorelines, wetlands) and private lands in the rural, suburban and urban context.

Exclusion: architecture and construction services, systems and policies (e515)

e525 **Housing services, systems and policies**
Services, systems and policies for the provision of shelters, dwellings or lodging for people.

e530 **Utilities services, systems and policies**
Services, systems and policies for publicly provided utilities, such as water, fuel, electricity, sanitation, public transportation and essential services.

Exclusion: civil protection services, systems and policies (e545)

e535 **Communication services, systems and policies**
Services, systems and policies for the transmission and exchange of information.

e540 **Transportation services, systems and policies**
Services, systems and policies for enabling people or
goods to move or be moved from one location to
another.

e545 **Civil protection services, systems and policies**
Services, systems and policies aimed at safeguarding
people and property.

Exclusion: utilities services, systems and policies (e530)

e550 **Legal services, systems and policies**
Services, systems and policies concerning the
legislation and other law of a country.

e555 **Associations and organizational services, systems
and policies**
Services, systems and policies relating to groups of
people who have joined together in the pursuit of
common, noncommercial interests, often with an
associated membership structure.

e560 **Media services, systems and policies**
Services, systems and policies for the provision of mass
communication through radio, television, newspapers
and internet.

e565   **Economic services, systems and policies**
Services, systems and policies related to the overall
system of production, distribution, consumption and
use of goods and services.

*Exclusion: social security services, systems and policies
(e570)*

e570   **Social security services, systems and policies**
Services, systems and policies aimed at providing
income support to people who, because of age,
poverty, unemployment, health condition or
disability, require public assistance that is funded
either by general tax revenues or contributory
schemes.

*Exclusion: economic services, systems and policies
(e565)*

e575   **General social support services, systems and policies**
Services, systems and policies aimed at providing
support to those requiring assistance in areas such as
shopping, housework, transport, self-care and care of
others, in order to function more fully in society.

*Exclusions: social security services, systems and policies
(e570); personal care providers and personal assistants
(e340); health services, systems and policies (e580)*

e580 **Health services, systems and policies**
Services, systems and policies for preventing and
treating health problems, providing medical
rehabilitation and promoting a healthy lifestyle.

*Exclusion: general social support services, systems and
policies (e575)*

e585 **Education and training services, systems and
policies**
Services, systems and policies for the acquisition,
maintenance and improvement of knowledge,
expertise and vocational or artistic skills. See
UNESCO's International Standard Classification of
Education (ISCED-1997).

e590 **Labour and employment services, systems and
policies**
Services, systems and policies related to finding
suitable work for persons who are unemployed or
looking for different work, or to support individuals
already employed who are seeking promotion.

*Exclusion: economic services, systems and policies
(e565)*

e595 **Political services, systems and policies**
Services, systems and policies related to voting,
elections and governance of countries, regions and
communities, as well as international organizations.

e598 Services, systems and policies, other specified

e599 Services, systems and policies, unspecified

ICF

Annexes

Annex 1

Taxonomic and terminological issues

The ICF classification is organized in a hierarchical scheme keeping in mind the following standard taxonomic principles:

- The components of Body Functions and Structures, Activities and Participation, and Environmental Factors are classified independently. Hence, a term included under one component is not repeated under another.

- Within each component, the categories are arranged in a stem–branch–leaf scheme, so that a lower-level category shares the attributes of the higher-level categories of which it is a member.

- Categories are mutually exclusive, i.e. no two categories at the same level share exactly the same attributes. However, this should not be confused with the use of more than one category to classify a particular individual's functioning. Such a practice is allowed, indeed encouraged, where necessary.

1. Terms for categories in ICF

Terms are the designation of defined concepts in linguistic expressions, such as words or phrases. Most of the terms over which confusion arises are used with common-sense meanings in everyday speech and writing. For example, impairment, disability and handicap are often used interchangeably in everyday contexts, although in the 1980 version of ICIDH these terms had stipulated definitions, which gave them a defined meaning. During the revision process, the term "handicap" was abandoned and "disability" has been used as an umbrella term for all three perspectives - body, individual and societal. Clarity and precision, however, are needed to define the various concepts, so that appropriate terms may be chosen to express each of the underlying concepts unambiguously. This is particularly important because ICF, as a written classification, will be translated into many languages. Beyond a common understanding of the concepts, it is also essential that an agreement be reached on the term that best reflects the content in each language. There may be many alternatives, and decisions should be made based on accuracy, acceptability, and overall usefulness. It is hoped that the usefulness of ICF will go in parallel with its clarity.

With this aim in mind, notes on some of the terms used in ICF follow:

Well-being is a general term encompassing the total universe of human life domains, including physical, mental and social aspects, that make up what can be called a "good life". Health domains are a subset of domains that make up the total universe of human life. This relationship is presented in the following diagram representing well-being:

Fig. 1   The universe of well-being

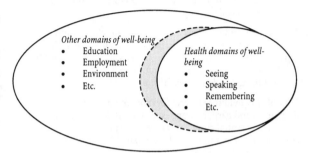

Health states and health domains: A health state is the level of functioning within a given health domain of ICF. Health domains denote areas of life that are interpreted to be within the "health" notion, such as those which, for health systems purposes, can be defined as the primary responsibility of the health system. ICF does not dictate a fixed boundary between health and health-related domains. There may be a grey zone depending on differing conceptualizations of health and health-related elements which can then be mapped onto the ICF domains.

Health-related states and health-related domains: A health-related state is the level of functioning within a given health-related domain of ICF. Health-related domains are those areas of functioning that, while they have a strong relationship to a health condition, are not likely to be the primary responsibility of the health system, but rather of other systems contributing to overall well-being. In ICF, only those domains of well-being related to health are covered.

Health condition is an umbrella term for disease (acute or chronic), disorder, injury or trauma. A health condition may also include other circumstances such as pregnancy, ageing, stress, congenital anomaly, or genetic predisposition. Health conditions are coded using ICD-10.

Functioning is an umbrella term for body functions, body structures, activities and participation. It denotes the positive aspects of the interaction between an individual (with a health condition) and that individual's contextual factors (environmental and personal factors).

Disability is an umbrella term for impairments, activity limitations and participation restrictions. It denotes the negative aspects of the interaction between an individual (with a health condition) and that individual's contextual factors (environmental and personal factors).

Body functions are the physiological functions of body systems, including psychological functions. "Body" refers to the human organism as a whole, and thus includes the brain. Hence, mental (or psychological) functions are subsumed under body functions. The standard for these functions is considered to be the statistical norm for humans.

Body structures are the structural or anatomical parts of the body such as organs, limbs and their components classified according to body systems. The standard for these structures is considered to be the statistical norm for humans.

Impairment is a loss or abnormality in body structure or physiological function (including mental functions). Abnormality here is used strictly to refer to a significant variation from established statistical norms (i.e. as a deviation from a population mean within measured standard norms) and should be used only in this sense.

Activity is the execution of a task or action by an individual. It represents the individual perspective of functioning.

Activity limitations[17] are difficulties an individual may have in executing activities. An activity limitation may range from a slight to a severe deviation in terms of quality or quantity in executing the activity in a manner or to the extent that is expected of people without the health condition.

Participation is a person's involvement in a life situation. It represents the societal perspective of functioning.

Participation restrictions[18] are problems an individual may experience in involvement in life situations. The presence of a participation restriction is determined by comparing an individual's participation to that which is expected of an individual without disability in that culture or society.

Contextual factors are the factors that together constitute the complete context of an individual's life, and in particular the background against which health states are classified in ICF. There are two components of contextual factors: Environmental Factors and Personal Factors.

Environmental factors constitute a component of ICF, and refer to all aspects of the external or extrinsic world that form the context of an individual's life and, as such, have an impact on that person's functioning. Environmental factors include the physical world and its features, the human-made physical world, other people in different relationships and roles, attitudes and values, social systems and services, and policies, rules and laws.

Personal factors are contextual factors that relate to the individual such as age, gender, social status, life experiences and so on, which are not currently classified in ICF but which users may incorporate in their applications of the classification.

---

[17] "Activity limitation" replaces the term "disability" used in the 1980 version of ICIDH.

[18] "Participation restriction" replaces the term "handicap" used in the 1980 version of ICIDH.

Facilitators are factors in a person's environment that, through their absence or presence, improve functioning and reduce disability. These include aspects such as a physical environment that is accessible, the availability of relevant assistive technology, and positive attitudes of people towards disability, as well as services, systems and policies that aim to increase the involvement of all people with a health condition in all areas of life. Absence of a factor can also be facilitating, for example the absence of stigma or negative attitudes. Facilitators can prevent an impairment or activity limitation from becoming a participation restriction, since the actual performance of an action is enhanced, despite the person's problem with capacity.

Barriers are factors in a person's environment that, through their absence or presence, limit functioning and create disability. These include aspects such as a physical environment that is inaccessible, lack of relevant assistive technology, and negative attitudes of people towards disability, as well as services, systems and policies that are either nonexistent or that hinder the involvement of all people with a health condition in all areas of life.

Capacity is a construct that indicates, as a qualifier, the highest probable level of functioning that a person may reach in a domain in the Activities and Participation list at a given moment. Capacity is measured in a uniform or standard environment, and thus reflects the environmentally adjusted ability of the individual. The Environmental Factors component can be used to describe the features of this uniform or standard environment.

Performance is a construct that describes, as a qualifier, what individuals do in their current environment, and so brings in the aspect of a person's involvement in life situations. The current environment is also described using the Environmental Factors component.

Taxonomic and terminological issues

Fig. 2   Structure of ICF

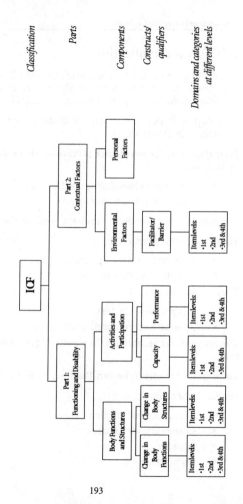

2. ICF as a classification

In order to understand the overall classification of ICF, it is important to understand its structure. This is reflected in the definitions of the following terms and illustrated in Fig. 2.

Classification is the overall structure and universe of ICF. In the hierarchy, this is the top term.

Parts of the classification are each of the two main subdivisions of the classification.

- Part 1 covers Functioning and Disability
- Part 2 covers Contextual Factors.

Components are each of the two main subdivisions of the parts.

The components of Part 1 are:

- Body Functions and Structures
- Activities and Participation.

The components of Part 2 are:

- Environmental Factors
- Personal Factors (not classified in ICF).

Constructs are defined through the use of qualifiers with relevant codes.

There are four constructs for Part 1 and one for Part 2.

For Part 1, the constructs are:

- Change in body function
- Change in body structure
- Capacity
- Performance

For Part 2, the construct is:

- Facilitators or barriers in environmental factors

Domains are a practical, meaningful set of related physiological functions, anatomical structures, actions, tasks, or areas of life. Domains make up the different chapters and blocks within each component.

Categories are classes and subclasses within a domain of a component, i.e. units of classification.

Levels make up the hierarchical order providing indications as to the detail of categories (i.e. granularity of the domains and categories). The first level comprises all the second-level items, and so on.

3. Definitions for ICF categories

Definitions are statements that set out the essential attributes (i.e. qualities, properties or relationships) of the concept designated by the category. A definition states what sort of thing or phenomenon the term denotes, and operationally, notes how it differs from other related things or phenomena.

During the construction of the definitions of the ICF categories, the following ideal characteristics of operational definitions, including inclusions and exclusions, were kept in mind:

- Definitions should be meaningful and logically consistent.

- They must uniquely identify the concept intended by the category.

- They must present essential attributes of the concept – both intentional (what the concept signifies intrinsically) and extensional (what objects or phenomena it refers to).

- They should be precise, unambiguous, and cover the full meaning of the term.

- They should be expressed in operational terms (e.g. in terms of severity, duration, relative importance, and possible associations).

- They should avoid circularity, i.e. the term itself, or any synonym for it, should not appear in the definition, nor should it include a term defined elsewhere using the first term in its definition.

- Where appropriate, they should refer to possible etiological or interactive factors.

- They must fit the attributes of the higher-ranking terms (e.g. a third-level term should include the general characteristics of the second-level category to which it belongs).

- They must be consistent with the attributes of the subordinate terms (e.g. the attributes of a second-level term cannot contradict those of third-level terms under it).

- They must not be figurative or metaphorical, but operational.

- They should make empirical statements that are observable, testable or inferable by indirect means.

- They should be expressed in neutral terms as far as possible, without undue negative connotation.

- They should be short and avoid technical terms where possible (with the exception of some Body Functions and Structures terms).

- They should have inclusions that provide synonyms and examples that take into account cultural variation and differences across the life span.

- They should have exclusions to alert users to possible confusion with related terms.

4. Additional note on terminology

Underlying the terminology of any classification is the fundamental distinction between the phenomena being classified and the structure of the classification itself. As a general matter, it is important to distinguish between the world and the terms we use to describe the world. For example, the terms 'dimension' or 'domain' could be precisely defined to refer to the world and 'component' and 'category' defined to refer only to the classification.

At the same time, there is a correspondence (i.e. a matching function) between these terms and it is possible that a wide variety of users may use these terms interchangeably. For more highly specialized requirements, for database construction and research modelling for example, it is essential for users to identify separately, and with a clearly distinct terminology, the elements of the conceptual model and those of the classification structure. Yet, it has been felt that the precision and purity that such an approach provides is not worth the price paid in a level of abstraction that might undermine the usefulness of the ICF, or more importantly to restrict the range of potential users of this classification.

Annex 2

Coding guidelines for ICF

ICF is intended for the coding of different health and health-related states.[19] Users are strongly recommended to read through the Introduction to ICF before studying the coding rules and guidelines. Furthermore, it is highly recommended that users obtain training in the use of the classification through WHO and its network of collaborating centres.

The following are features of the classification that have a bearing on its use.

1. Organization and structure

Parts of the Classification
ICF is organized into two parts.

Part 1 is composed of the following components:

- Body Functions and Body Structures
- Activities and Participation.

Part 2 is composed of the following components:

- Environmental Factors
- Personal Factors (currently not classified in the ICF).

---

[19] The disease itself should not be coded. This can be done using the International Statistical Classification of Diseases and Related Health Problems, Tenth Revision (ICD-10), which is a classification designed to permit the systematic recording, analysis, interpretation and comparison of mortality and morbidity data on diagnoses of diseases and other health problems. Users of ICF are encouraged to use this classification in conjunction with ICD-10 (see page 3 of Introduction regarding overlap between the classifications)

These components are denoted by prefixes in each code.

- *b* for Body Functions and
- *s* for Body Structures
- *d* for Activities and Participation
- *e* for Environmental Factors

The prefix *d* denotes the domains within the component of Activities and Participation. At the user's discretion, the prefix *d* can be replaced by *a* or *p*, to denote activities and participation respectively.

The letters *b*, *s*, *d* and *e* are followed by a numeric code that starts with the chapter number (one digit), followed by the second level (two digits), and the third and fourth level[20] (one digit each). For example, in the Body Functions classification there are these codes:

b2	Sensory functions and pain	(first-level item)
b210	Seeing functions	(second-level item)
b2102	Quality of vision	(third-level item)
b21022	Contrast sensitivity	(fourth-level item)

Depending on the user's needs, any number of applicable codes can be employed at each level. To describe an individual's situation, more than one code at each level may be applicable. These may be independent or interrelated.

In ICF, a person's health state may be assigned an array of codes across the domains of the components of the classification. The maximum number of codes available for each application is 34 at the chapter level (8 body functions, 8 body structures, 9 performance and 9 capacity codes), and 362 at the second level.

---

[20] Only the Body Functions and Body Structure classifications contain fourth-level items.

At the third and fourth levels, there are up to 1424 codes available, which together constitute the full version of the classification. In real-life applications of ICF, a set of 3 to 18 codes may be adequate to describe a case with two-level (three-digit) precision. Generally, the more detailed four-level version is intended for specialist services (e.g. rehabilitation outcomes, geriatrics, or mental health), whereas the two-level classification can be used for surveys and health outcome evaluation.

The domains should be coded as applicable to a given moment (i.e. as a snapshot description of an encounter), which is the default position. Use over time, however, is also possible in order to describe a trajectory over time or a process. Users should then identify their coding style and the time-frame that they use.

Chapters

Each component of the classification is organized into chapter and domain headings under which are common categories or specific items. For example, in the Body Functions classification, Chapter 1 deals with all mental functions.

Blocks

The chapters are often subdivided into "blocks" of categories. For example, in Chapter 3 of the Activities and Participation classification (Communication), there are three blocks: Communicating·Receiving (d310–d329), Communicating·Producing (d330–d349), and Conversation and using communication devices and techniques (d350–d369). Blocks are provided as a convenience to the user and, strictly speaking, are not part of the structure of the classification and normally will not be used for coding purposes.

Categories

Within each chapter there are individual two-, three- or four-level categories, each with a short definition and inclusions and exclusions as appropriate to assist in the selection of the appropriate code.

Definitions

ICF gives operational definitions of the health and health-related categories, as opposed to "vernacular" or layperson's definitions. These definitions describe the essential attributes of each domain (e.g. qualities, properties, and relationships) and contain information as to what is included and excluded in each category. The definitions also contain commonly used anchor points for assessment, for application in surveys and questionnaires, or alternatively, for the results of assessment instruments coded in ICF terms. For example, visual acuity functions are defined in terms of monocular and binocular acuity at near and far distances so that the severity of visual acuity difficulty can be coded as none, mild, moderate, severe or total.

Inclusion terms

Inclusion terms are listed after the definition of many categories. They are provided as a guide to the content of the category, and are not meant to be exhaustive. In the case of second-level items, the inclusions cover all embedded, third-level items.

Exclusion terms

Exclusion terms are provided where, owing to the similarity with another term, application might prove difficult. For example, it might be thought that the category "Toileting" includes the category "Caring for body parts". To distinguish the two, however, "Toileting" is excluded from category d520 "Caring for body parts" and coded to d530.

Other specified

At the end of each embedded set of third- or fourth-level items, and at the end of each chapter, are "other specified" categories (uniquely identified by the final code number 8). These allow for the coding of aspects of functioning that are not included within any of the other specific categories. When "other specified" is employed, the user should specify the new item in an additional list.

Unspecified

The last categories within each embedded set of third- or fourth-level items, and at the end of each chapter, are "unspecified" categories that allow for the coding of functions that fit within the group but for which there is insufficient information to permit the assignment of a more specific category. This code has the same meaning as the second- or third-level term immediately above, without any additional information (for blocks, the "other specified" and "unspecified" categories are joined into a single item, but are always identified by the final code number 9).

Qualifiers

The ICF codes require the use of one or more qualifiers, which denote, for example, the magnitude of the level of health or severity of the problem at issue. Qualifiers are coded as one, two or more numbers after a point. Use of any code should be accompanied by at least one qualifier. Without qualifiers codes have no inherent meaning (by default, WHO interprets incomplete codes as signifying the absence of a problem —xxx.00).
The first qualifier for Body Functions and Structures, the performance and capacity qualifiers for Activities and Participation, and the first qualifier for Environmental Factors all describe the extent of problems in the respective component.

All components are quantified using the same generic scale. Having a problem may mean an impairment, limitation, restriction or barrier, depending on the construct. Appropriate qualifying words as shown in brackets below should be chosen according to the relevant classification domain (where xxx stands for the second-level domain number):

xxx.0	NO problem	(none, absent, negligible,...)	0–4 %
xxx.1	MILD problem	(slight, low,...)	5–24 %
xxx.2	MODERATE problem	(medium, fair,...)	25–49 %
xxx.3	SEVERE problem	(high, extreme, ...)	50–95 %
xxx.4	COMPLETE problem	(total,...)	96–100 %
xxx.8	not specified		
xxx.9	not applicable		

Broad ranges of percentages are provided for those cases in which calibrated assessment instruments or other standards are available to quantify the impairment, capacity limitation, performance problem or environmental barrier/facilitator. For example, when "no problem" or "complete problem" is coded, this may have a margin of error of up to 5%. A "moderate problem" is defined as up to half of the scale of total difficulty. The percentages are to be calibrated in different domains with reference to population standards as percentiles. For this quantification to be used in a universal manner, assessment procedures have to be developed through research.

In the case of the Environmental Factors component, this first qualifier can also be used to denote the extent of positive aspects of the environment, or facilitators. To denote facilitators, the same 0–4 scale can be used, but the point is replaced by a plus sign: e.g. e110+2. Environmental factors can be coded either (i) in relation to each component; or (ii) without relation to each component (see section 3 below). The first style is preferable since it identifies the impact and attribution more clearly.

Additional qualifiers

For different users, it might be appropriate and helpful to add other kinds of information to the coding of each item. There are a variety of additional qualifiers that could be useful, as mentioned later.

Coding positive aspects

At the user's discretion coding scales can be developed to capture the positive aspects of functioning:

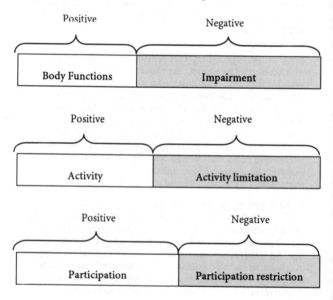

2. General coding rules

The following rules are essential for accurate retrieval of information for the various uses of the classification.

Select an array of codes to form an individual's profile

ICF classifies health and health-related states and therefore requires the assigning of a series of codes that best describe the profile of the person's functioning. ICF is not an "event classification" like ICD-10 in which a particular health condition is classified with a single code. As the functioning of a person can be affected at the body, individual and societal level, the user should always take into consideration all components of the classification, namely Body Functions and Structures, Activities and Participation, and Environmental Factors. Though it is impractical to expect that all the possible codes will be used for every encounter, depending on the setting of the encounter users will select the most salient codes for their purpose to describe a given health experience.

Code relevant information

Coded information is always in the context of a health condition. Although to use the codes it is not necessary to trace the links between the health condition and the aspects of functioning and disability that are coded, ICF is a health classification and so presumes the presence of a health condition of some kind. Therefore, information about what a person does or does not choose to do is not related to a functioning problem associated with a health condition and should not be coded. For example, if a person decides not to begin new relationships with his or her neighbours for reasons other than health, then it is not appropriate to use category d7200, which includes the actions of forming relationships. Conversely, if the person's decision is

linked to a health condition (e.g. depression), then the code
should be applied.

Information that reflects the person's feeling of involvement or
satisfaction with the level of functioning is currently not coded in
ICF. Further research may provide additional qualifiers that will
allow this information to be coded.

Only those aspects of the person's functioning relevant to a
predefined time-frame should be coded. Functions that relate to
an earlier encounter and have no bearing on the current
encounter should not be recorded.

Code explicit information

When assigning codes, the user should not make an inference
about the inter-relationship between an impairment of body
functions or structure, activity limitation or participation
restriction. For example, if a person has a limitation in
functioning in moving around, it is not justifiable to assume that
the person has an impairment of movement functions. Similarly,
from the fact that a person has a limited capacity to move around
it is unwarranted to infer that he or she has a performance
problem in moving around. The user must obtain explicit
information on Body Functions and Structures and on capacity
and performance separately. (In some instances, mental
functions for example, an inference from other observations is
required since the body function in question is not directly
observable.)

Code specific information

Health and health-related states should be recorded as
specifically as possible, by assigning the most appropriate ICF
category. For example, the most specific code for a person with
night blindness is b21020 "Light sensitivity". If, however, for
some reason this level of detail cannot be applied, the
corresponding "parent" code in the hierarchy can be used

instead (in this case, b2102 Quality of vision, b210 Seeing functions, or b2 Sensory functions and pain).

To identify the appropriate code easily and quickly, the use of the ICF Browser,[21] which provides a search engine function with an electronic index of the full version of the classification, is strongly recommended. Alternatively, the alphabetical index can be used.

3. Coding conventions for the Environmental Factors component

For the coding of environmental factors, three coding conventions are open for use:

Convention 1
Environmental factors are coded alone, without relating these codes to body functions, body structures or activities and participation.

Body functions	_____
Body structures	_____
Activities and Participation	_____
Environment	_____

Convention 2
Environmental factors are coded for every component.

Body functions _____	E code _____
Body structures _____	E code _____
Activities and Participation____	E code _____

---

[21] The ICF Browser in different languages can be downloaded from the ICF website: http://www.who.int/classification/icf

Convention 3

Environmental factors are coded for capacity and performance qualifiers in the Activities and Participation component for every item.

> Performance qualifier_____ E code _____
> Capacity qualifier_____ E code _____

4. Component-specific coding rules

4.1 Coding body functions

Definitions

Body functions are the physiological functions of body systems (including psychological functions). ***Impairments*** are problems in body function or structure as a significant deviation or loss.

Using the qualifier for body functions

Body functions are coded with one qualifier that indicates the extent or magnitude of the impairment. The presence of an impairment can be identified as a loss or lack, reduction, addition or excess, or deviation.

The impairment of a person with hemiparesis can be described with code b7302 Power of muscles of one side of the body:

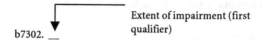

b7302. __   Extent of impairment (first qualifier)

Once an impairment is present, it can be scaled in severity using the generic qualifier. For example:

b7302.1	MILD impairment of power of muscles of one side of body	(5–24 %)
b7302.2	MODERATE impairment of power of muscles of one side of body	(25–49 %)
b7302.3	SEVERE impairment of power of muscles of one side of body	(50–95 %)
b7302.4	COMPLETE impairment of power of muscles of one side of body	(96–100 %)

The absence of an impairment (according to a predefined threshold level) is indicated by the value "0" for the generic qualifier. For example:

b7302.0   NO impairment in power of muscles of one side of body

If there is insufficient information to specify the severity of the impairment, the value "8" should be used. For example, if a person's health record states that the person is suffering from weakness of the right side of the body without giving further details, then the following code can be applied:

b7302.8   Impairment of power of muscles of one side of body, not specified

There may be situations where it is inappropriate to apply a particular code. For example, the code b650 Menstruation functions is not applicable for women before or beyond a certain age (pre-menarche or post-menopause). For these cases, the value "9" is assigned:

b650.9   Menstruation functions, not applicable

Structural correlates of body functions

The classifications of Body Functions and Body Structures are designed to be parallel. When a body function code is used, the user should check whether the corresponding body structure code is applicable. For example, body functions include basic human senses such as b210-b229 Seeing and related functions," and their structural correlates occur between s210 and s230 as "eye and related structures".

Interrelationship between impairments

Impairments may result in other impairments; for example, muscle power may impair movement functions, heart functions may relate to respiratory functions, perception may relate to thought functions.

Identifying impairments in body functions

For those impairments that cannot always be observed directly (e.g. mental functions), the user can infer the impairment from observation of behaviour. For example, in a clinical setting memory may be assessed through standardized tests, and although it is not possible to actually "observe" brain function, depending on the results of these tests it may be reasonable to assume that the mental functions of memory are impaired.

4.2 Coding body structures

Definitions

Body structures are anatomical parts of the body such as organs, limbs and their components. *Impairments* are problems in body function or structure as a significant deviation or loss.

Using qualifiers for coding body structures

Body structures are coded with three qualifiers. The first qualifier describes the extent or magnitude of the impairment, the second qualifier is used to indicate the nature of the change, and the third qualifier denotes the location of the impairment.

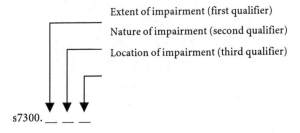

Extent of impairment (first qualifier)

Nature of impairment (second qualifier)

Location of impairment (third qualifier)

s7300. __ __ __

The descriptive schemes used for the three qualifiers are listed in Table 1.

Table 1. Scaling of qualifiers for body structures

First qualifier Extent of impairment	Second qualifier Nature of impairment	Third qualifier (suggested) Location of impairment
0 NO impairment 1 MILD impairment 2 MODERATE impairment 3 SEVERE impairment 4 COMPLETE impairment 8 not specified 9 not applicable	0 no change in structure 1 total absence 2 partial absence 3 additional part 4 aberrant dimensions 5 discontinuity 6 deviating position 7 qualitative changes in structure, including accumulation of fluid 8 not specified 9 not applicable	0 more than one region 1 right 2 left 3 both sides 4 front 5 back 6 proximal 7 distal 8 not specified 9 not applicable

4.3 Coding the Activities and Participation component

Definitions

Activity is the execution of a task or action by an individual.

Participation is involvement in a life situation.

Activity limitations are difficulties an individual may have in executing activities.

Participation restrictions are problems an individual may experience in involvement in life situations.

The Activities and Participation classification is a single list of domains.

Using the capacity and performance qualifiers

Activities and Participation is coded with two qualifiers: the *performance* qualifier, which occupies the first digit position after the point, and the *capacity* qualifier, which occupies the second digit position after the point. The code that identifies the category from the Activities and Participation list and the two qualifiers form the default information matrix.

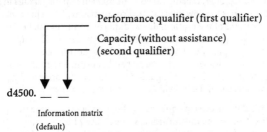

Performance qualifier (first qualifier)

Capacity (without assistance) (second qualifier)

d4500. __ __

Information matrix
(default)

The performance qualifier describes what an individual does in his or her current environment. Because the current environment brings in a societal context, performance as recorded by this qualifier can also be understood as "involvement in a life situation" or "the lived experience" of people in the actual context in which they live. This context includes the environmental factors – i.e. all aspects of the physical, social and attitudinal world. This features of the current environment can be coded using the Environmental Factors classification.

The capacity qualifier describes an individual's ability to execute a task or an action. This construct aims to indicate the highest probable level of functioning that a person may reach in a given domain at a given moment. To assess the full ability of the individual, one would need to have a "standardized" environment to neutralize the varying impact of different environments on the ability of the individual. This standardized environment may be: (a) an actual environment commonly used for capacity assessment in test settings; (b) in cases where this is not possible, an assumed environment which can be thought to have an uniform impact. This environment can be called the "uniform" or "standard" environment. Thus, the capacity construct reflects the environmentally adjusted ability of the individual. This adjustment has to be the same for all persons in all countries to allow international comparisons. To be precise, the features of the uniform or standard environment can be coded using the Environmental Factors component. The gap between capacity and performance reflects the difference between the impacts of the current and uniform environments and thus provides a useful guide as to what can be done to the environment of the individual to improve performance.

Typically, the capacity qualifier without assistance is used in order to describe the individual's true ability which is not enhanced by an assistance device or personal assistance. Since

the performance qualifier addresses the individual's current
environment, the presence of assistive devices or personal
assistance or barriers can be directly observed. The nature of the
facilitator or barrier can be described using the Environmental
Factors classification.

Optional qualifiers

The third and fourth (optional) qualifiers provide users with the
possibility of coding capacity with assistance and performance
without assistance.

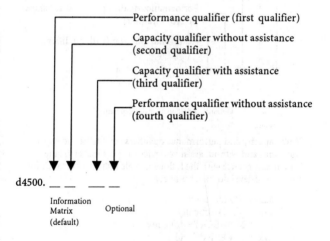

Additional qualifiers

The fifth digit position is reserved for qualifiers that may be developed in the future, such as a qualifier for involvement or subjective satisfaction.

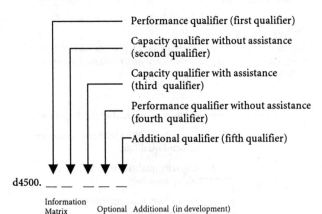

Performance qualifier (first qualifier)

Capacity qualifier without assistance (second qualifier)

Capacity qualifier with assistance (third qualifier)

Performance qualifier without assistance (fourth qualifier)

Additional qualifier (fifth qualifier)

d4500. _ _ _ _ _

Information Matrix (default)   Optional   Additional (in development)

Both capacity and performance qualifiers can further be used both with and without assistive devices or personal assistance, and in accordance with the following scale (where xxx stands for the second-level domain number):

    xxx.0 NO difficulty
    xxx.1 MILD difficulty
    xxx.2 MODERATE difficulty
    xxx.3 SEVERE difficulty
    xxx.4 COMPLETE difficulty
    xxx.8 not specified
    xxx.9 not applicable

When to use the performance qualifier and the capacity qualifier

Either qualifier may be used for each of the categories listed. But the information conveyed in each case is different. When both qualifiers are used, the result is an aggregation of two constructs, i.e.:

$$d4500.\ 2\ \_$$

d4500. 2 1 $\longrightarrow$

$$d4500.\_\ 1$$

If only one qualifier is used, then the unused space should not be filled with .8 or .9, but left blank, since both of these are true assessment values and would imply that the qualifier is being used.

Examples of the application of the two qualifiers

d4500 Walking short distances

For the *performance qualifier*, this domain refers to getting around on foot, in the person's current environment, such as on different surfaces and conditions, with the use of a cane, walker, or other assistive technology, for distances less than 1 km. For example, the performance of a person who lost his leg in a work-related accident and since then has used a cane but faces moderate difficulties in walking around because the sidewalks in the neighbourhood are very steep and have a very slippery surface can be coded:

d4500.3 _ moderate restriction in performance of walking short
            distances

For the *capacity qualifier*, this domain refers to the an individual's ability to walk around without assistance. In order to neutralize the varying impact of different environments, the ability may be assessed in a "standardized" environment. This standardized environment may be: (a) an actual environment commonly used for capacity assessment in test settings; or (b) in cases where this is not possible, an assumed environment which can be thought to have an uniform impact. For example, the true ability of the above-mentioned person to walk without a cane in a standardized environment (such as one with flat and non-slippery surfaces) will be very limited. Therefore the person's capacity may be coded as follows:

   d4500._ 3 severe capacity limitation in walking short distances

Users who wish to specify the current or standardized environment while using the performance or capacity qualifier should use the Environmental Factors classification (see coding convention 3 for Environmental Factors in section 3 above).

4.4 Coding environmental factors

Definitions

Environmental Factors make up the physical, social and attitudinal environment in which people live and conduct their lives.

Use of Environmental Factors

Environmental Factors is a component of Part 2 (Contextual Factors) of the classification. Environmental factors must be considered for each component of functioning and coded according to one of the three conventions described in section 3 above.

Environmental factors are to be coded from the perspective of the person whose situation is being described. For example, kerb cuts without textured paving may be coded as a facilitator for a wheelchair user but as a barrier for a blind person.

The qualifier indicates the extent to which a factor is a facilitator or a barrier. There are several reasons why an environmental factor may be a facilitator or a barrier, and to what extent. For facilitators, the coder should keep in mind issues such as the accessibility of a resource, and whether access is dependable or variable, of good or poor quality and so on. In the case of barriers, it might be relevant how often a factor hinders the person, whether the hindrance is great or small, or avoidable or not. It should also be kept in mind that an environmental factor can be a barrier either because of its presence (for example, negative attitudes towards people with disabilities) or its absence (for example, the unavailability of a needed service). The effects that environmental factors have on the lives of people with health conditions are varied and complex, and it is hoped that future research will lead to a better understanding of this interaction and, possibly, show the usefulness of a second qualifier for these factors.

In some instances, a diverse collection of environmental factors is summarized with a single term, such as poverty, development, rural or urban setting, or social capital. These summary terms are not themselves found in the classification. Rather, the coder should separate the constituent factors and code these. Once again, further research is required to determine whether there are clear and consistent sets of environmental factors that make up each of these summary terms.

First qualifier

The following is the negative and positive scale that denotes the extent to which an environmental factor acts as a barrier or a facilitator. Using a point alone denotes a barrier, whereas using the + sign instead denotes a facilitator, as indicated below:

xxx.0	NO barrier	xxx+0	NO facilitator
xxx.1	MILD barrier	xxx+1	MILD facilitator
xxx.2	MODERATE barrier	xxx+2	MODERATE facilitator
xxx.3	SEVERE barrier	xxx+3	SUBSTANTIAL facilitator
xxx.4	COMPLETE barrier	xxx+4	COMPLETE facilitator
xxx.8	barrier, not specified	xxx+8	facilitator, not specified
xxx.9	not applicable	xxx.9	not applicable

Annex 3

Acknowledgements

The development of ICF would not have been possible without the
extensive support of many people from different parts of the world who
have devoted a great amount of time and energy and organized
resources within an international network. While it may not be possible
to acknowledge them all here, leading centres, organizations and
individuals are listed below.

WHO Collaborating Centres for ICF

Australia: Australian Institute of Health and Welfare, GPO Box 570,
Canberra ACT 2601, Australia. Contact: Ros Madden.

Canada: Canadian Institute for Health Information, 377 Dalhousie
Street, Suite 200, Ottawa, Ontario KIN9N8, Canada. Contact: Helen
Whittome.

France: Centre Technique National d`Etudes et de Recherches sur
les Handicaps et les Inadaptations (CTNERHI), 236 bis, rue de Tolbiac,
75013 Paris, France. Contact: Marc Maudinet.

Japan: Japan College of Social Work, 3-1-30 Takeoka, Kiyose-city,
Tokyo 204-8555, Japan. Contact: Hisao Sato.

Netherlands: National Institute of Public Health and the
Environment, Department of Public Health Forecasting, Antonie van
Leeuwenhoeklaan 9, P.O. Box 1, 3720 BA Bilthoven, The Netherlands.
Contacts: Willem M. Hirs, Marijke W. de Kleijn-de Vrankrijker.

Nordic countries: Department of Public Health and Caring
Sciences, Uppsala Science Park, SE 75185 Uppsala, Sweden. Contact:
Björn Smedby.

United Kingdom of Great Britain and Northern Ireland: National
Health System Information Authority, Coding and Classification,
Woodgate, Loughborough, Leics LE11 2TG, United Kingdom. Contacts:
Ann Harding, Jane Millar.

USA: National Center for Health Statistics, Room 1100, 6525
Belcrest Road, Hyattsville MD 20782, USA. Contact: Paul J. Placek.

Task forces

International Task Force on Mental Health and Addictive, Behavioural,
Cognitive, and Developmental Aspects of ICIDH, Chair: Cille Kennedy,
Office of Disability, Aging and Long-Term Care Policy, Office of the
Assistant Secretary for Planning and Evaluation, Department of Health
and Human Services, 200 Independence Avenue, SW, Room 424E,
Washington, DC 20201, USA. Co-Chair: Karen Ritchie.

Children and Youth Task Force, Chair: Rune J. Simeonsson, Professor of
Education, Frank Porter Graham Child Development Center, CB # 8185,
University of North Carolina, Chapel Hill, NC 27599-8185, USA. Co-
Chair: Matilde Leonardi.

Environmental Factors Task Force, Chair: Rachel Hurst, 11 Belgrave
Road, London SW1V 1RB, England. Co-Chair: Janice Miller.

Networks

La Red de Habla Hispana en Discapacidades (The Spanish Network).
Coordinator: José Luis Vázquez-Barquero, Unidad de Investigacion en
Psiquiatria Clinical y Social Hospital Universitario "Marques de
Valdecilla", Avda. Valdecilla s/n, Santander 39008, Spain.

Council of Europe Committee of Experts for the Application of ICIDH,
Council of Europe, F-67075, Strasbourg, France. Contact: Lauri Sivonen.

Nongovernmental organizations

American Psychological Association, 750 First Street, N.E., Washington, DC 20002-4242, USA. Contacts: Geoffrey M. Reed, Jayne B. Lux.

Disabled Peoples International, 11 Belgrave Road, London SW1V 1RB, England. Contact: Rachel Hurst.

European Disability Forum, Square Ambiorix, 32 Bte 2/A, B-1000, Bruxelles, Belgium. Contact: Frank Mulcahy.

European Regional Council for the World Federation of Mental Health (ERCWFM), Blvd Clovis N.7, 1000 Brussels, Belgium. Contact: John Henderson.

Inclusion International, 13D Chemin de Levant, F-01210 Ferney-Voltaire, France. Contact: Nancy Breitenbach

Rehabilitation International, 25 E. 21st Street, New York, NY 10010, USA. Contact: Judith Hollenweger, Chairman, RI Education Commission, Institute of Special Education, University of Zurich, Hirschengraben 48, 8001 Zurich, Switzerland.

Consultants

A number of WHO consultants provided invaluable assistance in the revision process. They are listed below.

Elizabeth Badley, Jerome E. Bickenbach, Nick Glozier, Judith Hollenweger, Cille Kennedy, Jane Millar, Janice Miller, Jürgen Rehm, Robin Room, Angela Roberts , Michael F. Schuntermann, Robert Trotter II, David Thompson (editorial consultant)

Translation of ICF in WHO official languages

ICF has been revised in multiple languages taking English as a working language only. Translation and linguistic analysis have been integral part of the revision process. The following WHO collaborators have lead the translation, linguistic analyses, editorial review the WHO official languages. Other translations could be found on the WHO-web site: http://www.who.int/classification/icf.

Arabic

Translation and linguistic analysis: Adel Chaker, Ridha Limem, Najeh Daly, Hayet Baachaoui, Amor Haji, Mohamed Daly, Jamil Taktak, Saïda Douki

Editorial review carried out by WHO/EMRO: Kassem Sara, M. Haytham Al Khayat, Abdel Aziz Saleh

Chinese

Translation and linguistic analysis: Qiu Zhuoying (co-ordinator), Hong Dong, Zhao Shuying, Li Jing, Zhang Aimin, Wu Xianguang, Zhou Xiaonan

Editorial review carried out by WHO Collaborating Centre in China and WHO/WPRO: Dong Jingwu, Zhou Xiaonan and Y.C. Chong

French

Translation and linguistic analysis carried out by WHO Geneva:Pierre Lewalle

Editorial review carried out by WHO Collaborating Centres in France and Canada: Catherine Barral and Janice Miller

Russian

Translation and linguistic analysis: G. Shostka (Co-ordinator), Vladimir Y. Ryasnyansky, Alexander V. Kvashin, Sergey A. Matveev, Aleksey A. Galianov

Editorial review carried out by WHO Collaborating Centre in Russia: Vladimir K. Ovcharov

Spanish
Translation, linguistic analysis, editorial review by the Collaborating
Centre in Spain in collaboration with La Red de Habla Hispana en
Discapacidades (The Spanish Network) and WHO/PAHO: J. L.
Vázquez-Barquero (Co-ordinator), Ana Díez Ruiz, Luis Gaite Pindado,
Ana Gómez Silió, Sara Herrera Castanedo, Marta Uriarte Ituiño, Elena
Vázquez Bourgon Armando Vásquez, María del Consuelo Crespo, Ana
María Fossatti Pons, Benjamín Vicente, Pedro Rioseco, Sergio Aguilar
Gaxiola, Carmen Lara Muñoz, María Elena Medina Mora, María Esther
Araujo Bazán, Carlos Castillo-Salgado, Roberto Becker, Margaret
Hazlewood

Individual participants in the revision process

Over 1800 individuals in 65 WHO member states participated actively in
the revision process. A detailed list of the participants can be found in
the Annex 10 in the ICF Full Version.

Organisations of the United Nations system

International Labour Organization (ILO)
Susan Parker

United Nations Children's Fund (UNICEF)
Habibi Gulbadan

United Nations Statistical Division
Margarat Mbogoni
Joann Vanek

United Nations Statistical Institute for Asia and the Pacific
Lau Kak En

United Nations Economic and Social Commission for Asia
and Pacific
Bijoy Chaudhari

World Health Organization

Regional Offices

> Africa: C. Mandlhate
>
> Americas (Pan American Health Organisation): Carlos Castillo-Salgado, Roberto Becker, Margaret Hazlewood, Armando Vázquez
>
> Eastern Mediterranean: A. Mohit, Abdel Aziz Saleh, Kassem Sara, M. Haytham Al Khayat
>
> Europe: B. Serdar Savas, Anatoli Nossikov
>
> South-East Asia: Than Sein, Myint Htwe
>
> Western Pacific: R. Nesbit, Y.C. Chong

Headquarters

Various departments at WHO headquarters were involved in the revision process. Individual staff members who contributed to the revision process are listed below with their departments are listed below.

> M. Argandoña, formerly of Department of Substance Abuse
>
> Z. Bankowski, Council for International Organizations of Medical Sciences
>
> J.A. Costa e Silva, formerly Division of Mental Health and Prevention of Substance Abuse
>
> S. Clark, Department of Health Information, Management and Dissemination
>
> C. Djeddah, Department of Injuries and Violence Prevention
>
> A. Goerdt, formerly of Department of Health Promotion ·
>
> M. Goracci, formerly of Department of Injury Prevention and Rehabilitation

M. A. Jansen, formerly of Department of Mental Health and Substance Dependence

A. L'Hours, Global Programme on Evidence for Health Policy

A. Lopez, Global Programme on Evidence for Health Policy

J. Matsumoto, Department of External Cooperation and Partnerships

C. Mathers, Global Programme on Evidence for Health Policy

C. Murray, Global Programme on Evidence for Health Policy

H. Nabulsi, formerly of IMPACT

E. Pupulin, Department of Management of Noncommunicable Diseases

C. Romer, Department of Injuries and Violence Prevention

R. Sadana, Global Programme on Evidence for Health Policy

B. Saraceno, Department of Mental Health and Substance Dependence

A. Smith, Department of Management of Noncommunicable Diseases

J. Salomon, Global Programme on Evidence for Health Policy

M. Subramanian, formerly of World Health Reporting

M. Thuriaux, formerly of Division of Emerging and other Communicable Diseases

B. Thylefors, formerly of Department of Disability/Injury Prevention and Rehabilitation

M. Weber, Department of Child and Adolescent Health and Development

Sibel Volkan and Grazia Motturi provided administrative and secretarial support.

Can Çelik, Pierre Lewalle, Matilde Leonardi, Senda Bennaissa and Luis Prieto carried out specific aspects of the revision work.

Somnath Chatterji, Shekhar Saxena, Nenad Kostanjsek and Margie Schneider carried out the revision based on all the inputs received.

T. Bedirhan Üstün managed and coordinated the revision process and the overall ICF project.